# I Beat Cancer

**Bernice Wallin**
with Fred Wallin

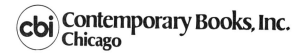

**cbi** Contemporary Books, Inc.
Chicago

**Library of Congress Cataloging in Publication Data**

Wallin, Bernice.
    I beat cancer.

    1. Breast—Cancer—Biography.    2. Wallin, Bernice.
I. Title.    [DNLM: 1. Neoplasms—Personal narratives.
QZ201 W211i]
RC280.B8W34        616.9′94′490924 [B]        77-83923
ISBN 0-8092-7736-0

Published by Contemporary Books, Inc.
180 North Michigan Avenue, Chicago, Illinois 60601
Manufactured in the United States of America
Library of Congress Catalog Card Number: 77-83923
International Standard Book Number: 0-8092-7736-0

Published simultaneously in Canada by
Beaverbooks
953 Dillingham Road
Pickering, Ontario L1W 1Z7
Canada

# *Foreword*

Immunotherapy as a means of treating cancer in humans has only recently developed a sufficient scientific basis to be accepted as a new means of treatment. An organized attempt by Dr. William Coley around the turn of the century, based on observations of cancer patients with bacterial infections living longer than those without infections, led him to develop a substance, named Coley toxin, from cultures of bacteria grown in the laboratory. Administration of this material to cancer patients was helpful to many but not to all. The lack of sufficient understanding of immunology made him unable to explain the lack of effectiveness in others and prevented further use of this material for those who would benefit. Today we know that both the strength of the substance and the immunological condition of the patient are critical for successful treatment.

About the same time, there was a great deal of work

being done to develop a vaccine against tuberculosis, which was a much more serious and widespread hazard in those days. Two French doctors, Albert Calmette and Camille Guerin, were the ones who were successful in solving this problem. They had struggled from 1904 until 1909 to weaken the strain of *Mycobacterium bovis* isolated by A. Nocard in 1904. By 1909, after repeated culturing in the laboratory through 230 transfers, they were able to demonstrate that the strain would no longer cause tuberculosis in animals. They continued their work, and in 1921 the vaccine was the first used in humans. In honor of their. work the vaccine was named Bacillus of Calmette-Guerin—BCG.

As an anti-tuberculosis vaccine, BCG has been very successful and over a half-billion people have been vaccinated with it since its introduction. Its safety record is unsurpassed by any other vaccine, and it is one of the most widely used vaccines in the world.

The first report of the use of the BCG vaccine in cancer appeared in Norway in 1935, but this report was not effective in inspiring others to do further work. Another report appeared in the Philippines in 1963; that also was not followed up. The basis for the modern use of BCG vaccine in cancer treatment was established, interestingly enough, by another Frenchman, Dr. George Mathe. In 1969 he published a report on the effective treatment of acute leukemia in humans with BCG. This report was firmly based on the many studies in animals and was the start of the current wave of immunotherapy of cancer with BCG.

Although there are other substances that can be used for the stimulation of the immune system, BCG vaccine has distinct advantages. Its long use as a human vaccine, the excellent safety record, and the rigid safety and efficacy tests that must be met for license use all serve as a starting point for the requirements for experimental use. BCG stimulates both the humoral immunity (antibodies) and cell-mediated immunity (white blood cells), so it is a general stimulator of any existing immunity that the patients may have. Many reports in the medical literature document the usefulness of BCG vaccine in the treatment of cancer and some reports have proposed its potential use for the prevention of cancer.

The victory over widespread cancer of Bernice Wallin is a success story that cannot be applied to all cancer patients. It is likely that BCG was able to stimulate her immune system to such an extent that it was directly responsible for the arresting of the progression of the disease and the establishment of remission. Even the most knowledgeable researchers · in the use of immunotherapy realize that Mrs. Wallin's case is still an exception to what can be expected because we still do not have sufficient understanding as to just why she had such a dramatic result. We are most gratified that Mrs. Wallin was helped by immunotherapy and we continue to hope and work diligently to improve immunotherapy so that as many patients as possible can be helped with this type of treatment. As Mrs. Wallin clearly explains in her book, equally important to the treatment is the fact that the condition of the patient's immune system is of critical importance in determining whether immunotherapy will be effective in any given patient. We do not know enough yet to determine which patients can be helped, but our current understanding of the response of the immune system is such that we can find indications of those patients who will benefit most through the treatment. Current investigations show that patients with a diminished immune response are helped much less but are helped to some degree by immunotherapy. It is the patients with a strong immune response still present at the beginning of treatment who will gain the maximum benefit.

As the value of BCG is realized, immunotherapy will be combined with surgery, radiation, and/or chemotherapy in an organized manner in which these various elements of treatment are orchestrated to make a harmonious whole in the treatment to successfully arrest or cure patients with cancer. Important for this harmony is that other treatments should not diminish the immune system for the immune stimulation that follows. Immunotherapy is still a relatively new treatment, but it is the success of patients such as Mrs. Wallin that gives us the hope and encouragement to pursue our goal of better medical treatment of all people with cancer and the dream of curing and even preventing cancer.

Ray G. Crispen, Ph.D.
*Director of the Institute of Tubercular Research*
*University of Illinois Medical Center*

# *Preface*

There are two stories in this book.

The first is an individual story, an uncommon chronicle of personal victory over a merciless foe against crushing odds. Bernice Wallin looked at the odds against her and decided to change them. Purely through courage, determination, and persistence, she succeeded. She is the indomitable human spirit, the phoenix rising from its ashes, an inspiration in our age of anti-heroes and organization men.

The second story concerns science and medicine in the twentieth century, and if Bernice Wallin's tale is a chronicle of the individual triumphant, the other story is not. Koch, Ehrlich, and Pasteur—they belong to the history books. Their methods relate to the twentieth century in the same manner as hoop skirts and Progressivism. Science and technology are complex now, so the single-handed medical breakthrough is rare. Many hands and talented minds participated in the revolution in cancer immunology that has occurred during the past two decades.

Insofar as the dearth of medical miracles reflects the complexity of nature, it is unavoidable; to the extent that it results from social custom, it is intolerable. Every cancer researcher can tell of projects unfunded, tantalizing leads left dangling. The pity is not that a modern Pasteur probably could not dream up a cure for cancer. It is that if he did so, *he would never be able to develop it.*

If the complexity of science has increased, the diversity of funding sources has dwindled. Most of the money comes from government. Cancer research teams pay tribute to Washington with modest progress reports, but great successes would threaten the reason for the existence of the research establishment. Nowadays researchers had better not be too imaginative because proposals whose outcome is not reasonably certain prior to the experimental work are likely to be turned down by the anonymous review panels. They had better not toot their own horns too enthusiastically—"unprofessional" use of the mass media is a sure route to oblivion.

The cancer bureaucracy, like the soon-to-be-created national health care bureaucracy, like any governmental body, possess a single *raison d'etre*—survival. Not curing cancer; not promoting health; just perpetuating itself, by perpetuating the *status quo.*

So it's not surprising that Bernice Wallin had to fight for her treatment, or that the treatment that helped her is still not widely available. It's not surprising that nobody seems to be coordinating the technological development of various experimental immunological findings for clinical applications; or that Mrs. Wallin's home state has powerful cancer laws that restrict treatment of the disease to conventional methods.

Medical science in the late twentieth century is a story of creativity thwarted, leads lost, technology with the satisfactions of *coitus interruptus.* It is superlative science pursued in the service of The System, and The System is a decerebrate brontosaurus that crashes through the darkness in aimless pursuit of its own existence.

Neither story in this book is complete. My hope is that the readers themselves can write a satisfying conclusion to the second story. To do so they can rely on the inspiration and the example provided by the first—the story of Bernice Wallin's triumph—for surely human stupidity is a more yielding foe than cancer.

Richard P. Huemer, M.D.
*Westlake Village, California*
*May 22, 1977*

# Chapter 1

Fɪʀsᴛ I ᴡᴀɴᴛ to roll some credits. But this is more than a dedication to my father, who died twenty-five years ago. It is a vital part of my story, because I feel I owe my life to the way my father raised me. If it weren't for Papa, that short, round, chubby man, with his fierce temper, who so terrified me as a child, I wouldn't be alive today. He never went to college, but I learned things from him I never learned from any of my professors. I have read Socrates, Nietzsche and Freud, but my most valuable education came from my father, who taught me how to survive.

Papa died in 1952, so he wasn't even around when I started my fight against cancer. The fight started in 1964, when I learned that my seven-year-old son had acute lymphatic leukemia. When cancer later invaded my own body, the fight continued—though it took some time for me to formulate the strategies and line up the battle fronts.

Mama was with me throughout the struggle, and she

gave me refuge and strength. But I was able to battle the disease only because Papa gave me the ammunition. It was Papa who taught me how to fight.

When I was a little girl, Papa told me that when I wanted something, I would often have to circumvent accepted procedure to get it. I would have to open doors that seemed locked and I'd have to reach the right people. He showed me how to get around rules—even if it meant breaking them. If he told me once, he told me a thousand times, "There are no such things as iron-clad rules. There are exceptions to every rule. Rules are made for two reasons: to bend or to break."

My father's rebellion against authority ran deep. He realized that there are two types of people in the world: those who give orders and those who take them. And, as far as my father was concerned, orders were not to be taken without being questioned. He did not trust people, especially people in power. Watergate would not have surprised him. He spoke in English and Yiddish, a language well suited to the expression of cynicism. "Don't accept people at face value," was my father's advice. "Don't trust people blindly. Motives should always be questioned." It was Papa who taught me never to take no for an answer. It was Papa who taught me how to survive.

Not that I'm putting my father up on a pedestal. Papa definitely had his faults. He wasn't exactly the most honest person. As a matter of fact, I think he had a touch of the gangster in him. But maybe it was the only way he knew of surviving.

We were a Jewish family living in Detroit, Michigan, during the depression of the thirties, when a lot of people weren't doing well financially. But Papa always managed. He owned a small clothing store, and when bills started piling up and the store wasn't exactly thriving, Papa found ways of putting food on the table. He was a hell of a good provider. So we tried not to question his ways.

He may have been a little dishonest, but I can't really

complain. Besides being a good provider, he was a good father, a thoughtful father. Every morning he used to get up and squeeze fresh orange juice for us. He delighted in doing that—scampering around the kitchen like a fat little kid, kissing Mama on the cheek, pouring the juice into each of our glasses.

When it snowed in winter, he used to pull us around in a big sleigh. Freezing cold and three feet of snow on the ground, but he'd be out there tugging and panting away, his big nose shining like a red light bulb.

And such a story teller, my father. I used to sit on his big, comfortable lap for hours, listening to stories about his childhood in Russia when anti-Semitism was very strong. There was one story that always fascinated me. When Papa was about ten years old, he saw a Cossack village marshal accept a bribe from a Jewish businessman who needed special permission to run his clothing store. The Jewish businessman was Papa's own father—my grandfather—and Papa remembered that scene in detail. I guess it taught him the power of money and the importance of getting to the right people. He was always telling us kids, "Just go right to the top. Forget the flunkies along the way and find the head man and go straight to him when you want something."

Papa wanted his kids to read, too. He wasn't an educated man himself, but he brought books home for us. There were encyclopedias, novels, biographies, anthologies—I mean, you name it and it was on our bookshelf.

Often when he caught me listening to music on the radio, he would toss a book to me and say, "Bossie, read. Get educated. Don't waste your time with music. Don't be a dummy."

I think he pressured me to read more than he did the others. I had two sisters and a brother, but I was the baby in the family, Papa's *mizinki*. And he wanted me to be really smart, to get ahead. He was always asking me questions about my homework and what I was learning in school, just checking to see if I was doing anything with my brain. He taught me to love learning, and reading became as necessary as eating, breathing, or sleeping. I gobbled up books voraciously.

As much as he loved and spoiled me, though, Papa frequently used me in his shadier money-making schemes. Abe Lincoln he was not. One of Papa's methods for keeping his family fed was the fraudulent insurance claim. He sued anyone he could—private parties or companies, it didn't matter. He even sued the city a few times.

One day he and I were walking down Woodward Avenue where some construction work was underway and Papa whispered to me, "Bossie, when we get to the curb, I want you to pretend you tripped in that crack over there."

Now, I was only five years old, but I knew he was going to sue somebody, because *sue* had been part of my vocabulary for a long time. And I knew I was going to be part of some grand scheme he had planned.

But I just couldn't fall. I was afraid I would hurt myself. And I knew a lot of people would see me fall and I didn't know if I could pull if off. So this time I didn't fall.

As we were crossing the street, Papa squeezed my hand hard and muttered, "So, what's the matter with you, stinker? You didn't hear me? I said fall! Now, when we get to the other side, you fall, you hear me? And you cry. Real loud."

But I didn't have to fall. He shoved me. And I cried, all right. But not because I hurt myself. I cried because I was so humiliated and so mad at Papa.

Papa was always falling himself and spraining something so he could sue somebody. I never saw a man with so many sprains in one body. And he got whiplashes in the most unlikely ways. I've heard that other failing businessmen in the thirties did the same kinds of things Papa did to get by, and I've always wondered why none of those insurance companies ever realized they were being taken.

But in our case, they never did. And with all his insurance claims, Papa became pretty familiar with doctors and lawyers. He wasn't impressed with them at all. Sometimes he'd just burst through our front door, ranting and raving about how some son-of-a-bitch doctor had tried to get a bigger share of the insurance money or how one of the lawyers had almost screwed up a deal by backing down or something.

Papa would stand in the middle of the living room floor, all red in the face, his big belly protruding about a half foot in front of him, and he'd put his hands on his hips, shake his head, and say, "I just can't believe it, these doctors. People treat 'em like gods, but I'm telling you, a doctor is a *mench vee alleh menchen* (a man like all men). Greedy, crooked, they have no right in the medical profession, some of 'em."

How Papa lived with himself, though, I don't know. I could see right through him, and sometimes I didn't like what I saw. As much as I adored him, there was much about him I could not admire.

His religious beliefs, for instance. If Papa's religion had had a label, it would have been Superstition, not Judaism. Every positive statement was punctuated with *"Kinehora,"* which, loosely translated, carries much the same meaning as "Knock on wood."

I'm not sure Papa actually believed in anything but himself. Yet he seemed to be constantly in fear of incurring God's wrath. So, to be on the safe side, he donned his *tefillen* and prayed at the right times. But as soon as he'd finished being righteous, he'd go right out and con someone. When I got old enough to really think about God, I finally realized that what Papa thought was religion was really just an assortment of superstition and rituals performed to hedge his bets, just in case such a being as God existed.

To avoid God's anger, for example, Papa believed one should not laugh too loudly, or display happiness. "Stop that laughing, Bossie," he would caution me when I acted especially happy, "or you will offend God and He will give you an evil eye or *tsuris*." Later in my life, when troubles started piling up, I wondered if I had flaunted my happiness too openly or laughed too loudly.

I'm sure it was Papa who loaded me with guilt. He blamed his kids for everything. There were four of us; Rosie, Elvin, Sally, and I. If business was bad at the store, if he lost a law suit, if he missed a bus, if a cat crossed his path, he'd point an accusing finger in our direction and scream at us. And yet, as often as Papa screamed at us, for getting Bs instead of As, for arguing among ourselves, or for whatever annoyed him, he never laid a finger on us. But every time he threatened, we were sure that that would be the time he would really smack us and we were all frightened enough to obey.

I've lived with guilt practically all my life, from childhood through adulthood and right up to the present. As a parent, if I wasn't doing something for my children I felt guilty. I mean, I loved doing things for them, but sometimes I think I did too much. And I'm sure it was Papa's legacy of guilt that made me feel it was necessary.

When I was a child, I thought that there was no question Papa couldn't answer, no problem he couldn't resolve. But as I got older, I rebelled a little. And I think Papa liked that.

I remember well the first time I challenged his authority. It was like taking my life into my hands, believe me, but I think Papa secretly liked my show of independence.

As a teenager I loved to dance—did the meanest jitterbug and rhumba in town. As a matter of fact, I still have quite a few trophies in my closet that I won in some dancing contests in the forties. I went dancing every night I got the chance, and Papa thought I went much too often.

One evening I was standing in front of the bathroom mirror getting ready to go out dancing. I had just hennaed my hair the night before. My hair was mousy brown and I wanted it auburn. Papa thought that was fine; if you want something, go get it. He had even helped me get the parts in the back I couldn't reach.

As I was primping away in front of the mirror, Papa came clomping down the hall. He stopped at the bathroom door and stood watching me.

"So, dancing again tonight, Bossie?"

"Yes, Papa, there's a contest tonight and I'm gonna win again," I bubbled.

He grew stern and his eyes glinted at me. "You go dancing too much, Bossie. What about your homework?"

"Oh, I'll do it this weekend, Papa, but this is Friday, and no one does homework on Friday night."

"And why not? What's wrong with exercising your brain on Friday night instead of your legs?"

"Oh, nothing's wrong unless you'd rather be dancing," I replied flippantly. "I feel like I'm being born again when I'm dancing."

"Born, smorn. You and your dancing. What's dancing? Nothing! Well, you can't go. I want you to stay home and do your homework," he said.

I couldn't believe my ears. I could see him in the mirror behind me and his eyes were very narrow. I felt that he was testing me.

"I've already made plans, Papa," I said. "So I have to go."

"Break the plans," he replied evenly.

Then I got mad. I whirled around and faced him. "Papa, I'm going to go dancing," I told him. "So you can just forget it."

We stared at each other a few minutes, and I could have sworn he was going to smile at me. His lips twitched a little. His right eye squinted at me.

But he just walked away.

I did go dancing that night, too. He didn't try to stop me. Never said a thing about it. And that was that. I think he was kind of proud of me.

Those are the things my father taught me. His was not always the best way to teach a kid, I suppose. But his lessons about going to the top and cutting through red tape to get what you want, about questioning authority, about sticking to your guns when you want something, about the value of knowledge—those lessons were ammunition in my battle against cancer. If Papa hadn't taught me those things, I'd probably be dead right now.

Five years ago, when breast cancer had spread to my bones and ribs, doctors said they didn't have much hope for me. They pulled the theoretical sheet over my head, told me there was no cure, and sent me home.

By that time I had been through the tragedy of my son's leukemia, and I had lost both my breasts. I was almost defeated at that point, almost beaten. But my rebellious nature—a product of Papa's teachings—kept me from complete surrender. I put up one last snarling good struggle. I had to be a little pushy at times. I had to yell at a few doctors, insist on my rights as a patient, and cut through a lot of red tape.

But I won my battle. And if I can tell how I beat cancer, perhaps I can provide some shortcuts for other cancer victims. Maybe I can open some doors and minds. Here's my story, in the name of my son Gary, who also suffered, and in the name of my father, David Sallan, who taught me how to survive.

# Chapter 2

I LOOK BACK WITH WONDER on the days before cancer invaded my life. It seems impossible that living could ever have been normal, let alone truly joyful. But if I dredge back far enough and somehow manage to forget all the pain and heartache of the last ten or twelve years, I realize that those days—before all the sickness and death—were indeed filled with joy.

When my youngest son, Gary, came along, he closed the gap left in our family circle by my husband, Jack. Jack spent his days working and his nights gambling in Gardena, a city fifteen miles from our home where gambling is legal. His main goal in life was to make the "Big Win." Because he was so seldom at home, the four boys and I made up the family unit.

It wasn't easy to be both parents to a bunch of boys. I worked part-time as a medical typist to make a little money for things Jack's salary wouldn't cover. Mama was living with us about three weeks out of every month, so I did have some help. But raising the kids and working in the evenings took all my energy. Nevertheless, I must admit I was in my glory as a mother. I loved my sons and I took motherhood very seriously.

I think the best year of my life must have been 1963. That was the year before we found out Gary had leukemia. All my sons seemed pretty healthy, we were closer than ever before, and Gary was becoming a little man. He seemed to mature faster than my other sons did, emotionally and intellectually. I've often wondered if his rush to manhood was somehow portentous.

By that time, Gary had perfected his Elvis Presley imitation. He was five years old, and Elvis was his idol. His eight-year-old brother, David, used to help him with the Elvis routines, because he was an avid Presley fan too. For that matter, all five of us were nuts for Elvis—like a bunch of teeny boppers—crazy.

One afternoon I found Gary doing his Elvis routine. He was standing in front of the record player in his room, his tawny brown locks pulled over his forehead, his hips swaying, lip-syncing his favorite Elvis song, "Return to Sender." I stood in the doorway watching.

He looked up and smiled at me. "Hi, Mom."

"So what're you up to, Elvis?"

"Mark's going-away party is this afternoon and he said I could be the entertainment," Gary told me.

"The entertainment?" I laughed.

"Yeah! Wanna see?"

I sat on the bed and he started the record over.

He closed his eyes, put his hands out in front of him, palms down, wiggled his hips, and didn't miss a beat.

I could hardly restrain my laughter. It was just so funny to see a five-year-old kid trying to be sexy. But if a five-year-old kid *could* be sexy, I told myself, he was.

When the record was over, he asked me to watch a few other routines. Then I helped him get dressed for the party.

He wanted to wear a suit and tie to the party, though I

told him Elvis hardly ever performed in a suit and tie. But he insisted. He was always trying to look so grown up.

He was a handsome kid. A show-stopper like my other three. Thick brown hair, olive complexion, a turned-up nose, and sparkling black cherry eyes. People were always stopping me to tell me how good-looking he was. Of course I believed them. Why shouldn't I? I could see for myself he was gorgeous.

When the party was over later that afternoon, Gary came home a little dejected. The kids had made fun of his Elvis impression. He'd probably fantasized a rapt audience and found instead a bunch of disinterested, rowdy five-year-olds.

I took him out in the backyard to help me work in the garden. He had his own vegetable garden out there and loved working in the earth and watching things grow.

"Well, don't worry about it, sweetheart," I tried to comfort him as we sat in the dirt sorting through the weeds. "When you grow up you can be a singer just like Elvis if you want to."

"He's so neat," Gary mumbled.

"He sure is."

"Yeah. Man, I wanna be just like him. Re-turn to sen-dah, doo de doo de doo, add-ress un-known, doo de doo de doo."

"Well, I think you act just like him."

"Really? Just like him?"

"Sure."

That seemed to make him happy. "Mom," he said, yanking viciously at the weeds, "could I be an Indian Guide?"

"A what?"

"An Indian Guide. It's a club. Joey and his dad are in it and I wanna be in it, too. Can I?"

"Well sure you can, honey, who do I call to get you in it?"

"Daddy has to call."

"Daddy? why Daddy?"

"The dads have to be in it with the kids," he said. "But it's a lot of fun. Maybe Daddy would like it. They go camping and play softball and they go backpacking. What's backpacking, Mommy?"

My heart was slowly sinking. If dads had to be in it, Gary might as well forget it. "Backpacking is like hiking," I told him. "But maybe you'd rather wait a year or two and get into Cub Scouts. Like your brothers were. Remember? When I was den mother? They went camping and hiking and all those things. Why don't you wait till then?"

"No, I wanna be an Indian Guide. You should see the outfits they get to wear, Mommy. Can I be in it?"

. "Sounds to me like you'd better ask your father," I told Gary. But I knew Jack would say no. He was no good at that kind of thing. Not that he was ever cruel or cold to the boys. He just didn't want to spend any time away from his gambling.

A few days later, Gary took the matter up with Jack. It was a silvery gray morning, cold and bleak. Gary and I woke up almost simultaneously every morning. I could hear him stirring in his bed a few moments after I'd opened my eyes.

I waited—two or three minutes—and he came padding down the hall to our room.

"Hi, angel," I whispered as he crawled into bed between Jack and me. He'd been doing that almost every morning since he could walk.

His little feet and hands were icy. He snuggled up next to me and said, "Morning, Mommy."

"The giant's still asleep," I whispered. It was a game we played. Jack was the sleeping giant and we had to be careful not to wake him up or he would eat us all gone.

I tickled Gary and he giggled.

"Shhh! You'll wake him up," I warned.

"Should I ask him about the Indian Guides?"

"This morning?"

"Yeah!"

"You sure you want a giant to be an Indian Guide with you?" I teased.

"Oh Mom!" he said. Then he turned over and put his hand on Jack's shoulder.

"Morning, son," Jack mumbled.

"Hey Dad, guess what," Gary began enthusiastically. "Wanna be an Indian Guide with me?"

Jack sat up slowly, swung his legs out of bed and sat there, his back to us. He ran his hand through his hair and got up, as if he hadn't even heard Gary.

Gary scrambled out of bed and followed his father down the hall to the bathroom. I couldn't hear the conversation but I could see when Gary walked back into the bedroom that Jack had refused. "He doesn't want to," he said sadly.

"Well, that's okay, honey." I sat up in bed and motioned for him to crawl in next to me. He nestled against me, small and quiet and defeated.

I felt so bad for Gary. I wanted to scream at Jack. But it would have done no good. I had done all the begging and screaming I would ever do. There was just no way to get through to him any more. Jack would never change. Gambling was his life. It was an obsession that left him no time for anything else.

Like most men, Jack was away all day working. Away from the daily anxieties and problems that occur in a houseful of boys. When he came home from his butcher's job in a classy kosher-style meat market in Los Angeles, he'd smile and give us a cheery hello, but then he'd withdraw into silence. If I tried to discuss a problem, get his opinion, ask his advice, he'd say, "Do you have to tell me this now?" Perhaps he was right. Perhaps there was a better time to talk about things, but I've been looking for it for thirty years and haven't found it yet. We shared the same bed, the same car, and the same breakfast table. But that's all we shared.

I used to nag Jack about not spending any time with his sons, and sometimes he would break down and take us all to Kiddyland or to the zoo on a Sunday, but you could tell his heart wasn't in it. He'd hurry us through, take us out for a quick bite to eat, drop us off at home, and then make a mad dash for Gardena.

He actually considered gambling a business, and one with a future, at that. Most compulsive gamblers do. They enjoy winning and manage to enjoy losing almost as much. I eventually became resigned to it. Now I realize that gambling is a disease. Not as deadly as cancer, but almost as debilitating to the spirit. I don't nag Jack about his gambling any more. It would be like nagging someone for being sick.

Fred, my oldest son, was fifteen in 1963. He had a life of his own to lead, but he made time for his brothers when they needed him. They really adored Fred; he gave them someone to look up to.

Fred was a thinker and a doer, and he didn't let anything stop him when he wanted something. Some of Papa had lived on in my children.

One day Fred came to me and asked, "Mom, who owns the airwaves?"

Good question. I thought I remembered reading that the public owned the airwaves and told him so.

"That's what I figured. So, if the public owns the airwaves, then why can't I watch CBS's game of the week with 'good old Dizzy Dean' doing the announcing? We used to watch it all the time on TV. Remember? Now, all of a sudden it's not on anymore."

"That's so people will go to the games, Fred, and not stay home and watch the games on television. It's big business, honey—just a matter of money, that's all."

"I know. And that's not fair. San Diego gets the games. And I'm going to get them too. Watch me!"

After reading up on the subject, he went to the electronics store six blocks from our house and bought a directional antenna. He brought it home and explained his plan to me.

Jack was at work. Paul and David were at the park

playing ball, so Gary and I were the only ones there to help him. Gary was fascinated by all the wires and screws, and his eyes lit up when Fred told him we'd soon have the Dodgers playing ball in our living room.

We pulled a ladder out of the garage and I followed Fred up to the roof. That was a major effort for me, because I have a fear of heights, but I was so proud of Fred and so anxious to see him pull off his caper that I followed him up the ladder and helped him put up the antenna.

Gary had pleaded with us to let him come up, too, but I said no. So he waited below, yelling up at us every two or three minutes, jumping around on our lawn and telling all the passers-by that we were going to get the Dodger games at our house.

When it was time to come down, I realized how high up in the air I was and nearly passed out.

"C'mon, Mom, let me help you," said Fred, holding out his hand.

"I can't do it, Fred," I said. "I can't."

"What do you mean, you can't do it? You have to do it," he said. "What are you going to do, live up here?"

"I don't know." I looked down at our front yard and I felt as if I were standing at the top of a skyscraper. "Oh, I can't, Fred," I said.

"Mom, your face is white as a sheet. Are you . . ."

"Gary!" I yelled down. "Gary, go call the fire department!"

"Mom, don't be ridiculous," said Fred.

"I can't come down by myself," I trembled.

"Well here, I'm going to go down and . . ." He started down the ladder.

"No, don't leave me!" I panicked. "Hey, Gary!"

"What, Mom?" Gary yelled up at me, his hands cupped around his mouth.

"Go call the fire department!" I yelled. "Tell them there's a lady stuck on your roof!"

We finally made Gary understand that we weren't

kidding and he went in to call the fire department. That was delightful for him, especially when the big red fire truck pulled up to our house with its lights flashing.

When I finally got down and everything was back to normal, we found that the San Diego television station came in clear as a bell.

"Stupid antenna specialist said it was impossible!" Fred gloated.

And Gary couldn't stop telling everyone that his oldest brother had performed a miracle. To him, Fred was the greatest.

Gary adored his older brothers and they felt the same way about him. They thought he was terrific. They thought he had "guts." Only they called it *chutzpah.* "Gary's got *chutzpah,"* they were always saying.

I guess you could say Gary knew how to manipulate people. Only "manipulation" isn't such a good word, because people loved it when Gary turned on the charm, even if it was to get something he wanted. Papa would have been proud of Gary.

We had a next-door neighbor—Laurie was her name— who was a landscape artist. She had the most gorgeous lawn on our block—all ivy, three-feet-tall ivy, which she manicured daily and sprayed diligently with enormous doses of DDT. And her rose gardens were perfection.

Whenever the kids' baseballs went into her yard, Gary volunteered to go romping through the ivy after them. This took a good deal of bravery, since Laurie often came out and yelled at him for messing up her ivy. I used to cringe whenever I saw him diving around in all that DDT, but I figured it probably wouldn't hurt him, and besides, he was having such fun.

One day David came dragging into the kitchen, all upset.

"What's the matter? Your ball go into Laurie's yard again?" I asked him.

He nodded and slumped down at the kitchen table.

"Our last ball, too," he sighed. "She keeps them if Gary doesn't get 'em first."

"She come out and yell at you?"

"Yeah." Then he puffed himself up. "You boys, I've told you a million times not to play ball around here," he mimicked her. "Her and her roses."

A few minutes later Paul came into the house and opened the door of the refrigerator, looking for something to eat. He was eleven at the time and had the appetite of three grown men. "Gary's at Laurie's," he said nonchalantly.

"At Laurie's? What's he doing there?" I asked.

"Said he was going to get our ball," Paul said, grabbing an apple. "If anyone can do it, he can. He could talk a frog out of its warts."

I took the apple from Paul's hand and placed it back in the refrigerator. "Lunch will be soon," I told him. "Just hang on."

He walked over to the back door and looked over at Laurie's house. "Look at him standing there," he said, peering through the curtains. "C'mere, Mom."

Gary was standing at her door talking to Laurie and within minutes he disappeared inside her house.

"Did you see him? That little con artist," Paul said with a grin.

A half hour later Gary came charging through our back door with the ball in his hand. "Got it!" he cried, holding it out victoriously.

"All *right!*" yelled Davey. "Gary, you've got *chutzpah,* ya know?"

"How'd you do it, you stinker?" asked Paul, ruffling Gary's hair. He was clearly proud of his little brother.

Gary shrugged. "Just asked her for it," he said.

"What did she say?" I wanted to know.

"Oh nothing. She gave me some coffee and cookies."

"Coffee?" I said. "What does she think you are, an old man?"

"I like coffee," he told me. "So she gave me some. It was real good. She put a bunch of cream and sugar in it."

"And then she gave you your ball? Just like that?"

"Yeah. I told her we were sorry and everything and she just said it was okay and gave me back the ball. She's a pretty nice lady. Once you get to know her," he said. "She wants me to come back sometime. Could I have some coffee for lunch, Mom?"

"For lunch?" I laughed. "I hardly think so, *mizinik*." I called Fred into the kitchen and sat them all down at the table. "Now what does everyone want for lunch?" I asked.

"Hot dog," said Fred.

"I'll have peanut butter and jelly, Mom," said David.

"How about you, Paul?"

"Oh, I don't know. Got any salami?"

"Sure, I think so.

"Gary, what do you want?"

"Aw, I'm not hungry, Mom," he said. "Just a cup of coffee would be fine."

"G-a-r-y."

"How 'bout tuna fish?"

I then proceeded to race around the kitchen like a short order cook, fixing each one exactly what he wanted. I know it may sound ridiculous, but yes, I catered to my sons. They got what they wanted, even if it meant fixing four separate meals at each mealtime. But I felt that was my job—to pamper them.

Some people say I spoiled my kids. I guess I did. I let my house go so I could chauffeur them around town, be involved in their activities, play games with them. I'm sure a lot of the neighbors thought me a harried, crazy mother. "You know Bernice Wallin, the chicken soup mother up the street. Spoils her kids rotten. Hope they turn out okay."

But I didn't care what people said. We didn't have Jack, my kids and me. But we had each other. We all had something to give each other, each in his own way. Fred, with his soulful brown eyes, always had words of wisdom to give; Paul, the driving, energetic one, gave us hope and optimism; David, the plodder, slow and deliberate, gave comfort and reliability; and Gary, the little imp with the delicious smile, gave joy.

I guess I spoiled Gary even more than I did the others. He was the baby in the family, my *mizinik,* as I had been Papa's *mizinki.* Gary was my fourth Caesarian section. When the nurse at the hospital put him into my arms, I gasped. He was that beautiful. Those huge black eyes darted around the room, alert and inquisitive, even at birth. He had a thatch of gold-brown hair and a perfectly turned up nose. A perfect nose. I smiled to myself. Thank you someone up there. He'll never need plastic surgery. I knew Gary would probably be my last child, so, okay, I spoiled him outrageously. But it was unavoidable. He was so special.

I'm not the only one who thought so. Others recognized it, too. Laurie told me after Gary died that he was one of the most special kids she had ever known.

Just to watch his unquenchable enthusiasm, his pleasure in a robin, a new leaf, the corn he planted that started to sprout, was such a joy. He would squinch his nose up with pleasure and my heart would say, "I'll never get enough of loving this child. I could die on the spot from loving him so much."

Okay, so you think he couldn't be as perfect as all that. You think some of the time he must have been a child like other children, whining, pouting, stubborn, demanding, irritable. And you're right, of course. He wasn't perfect. But I prefer to remember the good times. And I have to breathe life back into my son from time to time, because he must be remembered. He simply must.

I loved getting him off to school in the morning. We'd huddle over the furnace together to get warm first. Then he'd race off to get dressed while I fixed breakfast. He left the house almost every day wearing that silly tie, his hair slicked down with Vitalis, sauntering down the street to school.

Gary loved people and they loved him. I would fret and worry when he was late getting home from school. He had the habit of talking to anyone and everyone and I was afraid someone would steal him. When he did get home, we'd go over his school work, take long walks, tell each other monster stories, draw pictures, and play word games.

He was such a little *yenta,* my kid, you wouldn't believe. He never stopped talking. It was a nonstop conversation, especially the questions. He woke up at six with questions and fell into bed exhausted every night at seven with more questions.

And then at night I'd read him to sleep. He was such a good reader. His teacher told me he was a couple of years ahead of himself and they were thinking of skipping him a grade.

He'd sit up in bed all snug in his cowboy pajamas and listen attentively while I read. Sometimes he'd read a page and then I'd read a page. When he began to grow sleepy, he'd cuddle down beneath the blankets and listen to me read one of his favorite books, *Peter Pan.* I'd rub his neck as I read. Once in a while he'd look at me with his eyebrows knit in puzzlement and say something like, "Could that really happen, Mommy?" or "Is there really a place like that?" I remember one night he touched my cheek and said, "Now why didn't he want to grow up, Mommy? Peter Pan was nuts. I can't wait to grow up."

Had he grown up, I know Gary would have been kind and sensitive. He was always showing his love and devotion. He liked to make little presents and sometimes used his birthday money to buy me bottles of dimestore perfume.

So you must forgive me if I'm a little prejudiced. My son Paul was probably right when he told me I only think of Gary's being so great because he died. All I know is he did the most marvelous things for people, and I'll never forget them.

For our sixteenth wedding anniversary, for instance, Gary made plans for the whole family to go out for dinner. Somehow he managed to talk Jack out of gambling that evening. It was difficult to figure Jack out and though he never got involved in the lives of his children, I felt he was proud of them, especially Gary. He was a pushover for Gary. Jack agreed to celebrate at Gary's favorite restaurant—a barbecue place.

Our anniversary had lost its romantic aspect years before, but I was touched that my son was trying to make it special for me.

After we'd eaten our fill of barbecued beef and french fries, the waitress cleared away our dishes. Gary fidgeted and squirmed, his face glowing and his eyes darting nervously around the room.

Then suddenly we heard singing from the back of the restaurant.

"Happy anniversary to you."

Jack looked up, panic-stricken.

"Happy anniversary to you."

The singing was headed our way.

"Happy anniversary, Mr. and Mrs. Wallin."

There stood three waitresses and a bus boy at our table with a big chocolate cake, "Happy Anniversary" written across it.

"Happy anniversary to you!"

The whole restaurant applauded. Jack looked as if he wanted to die on the spot. I was delighted. And Gary was bubbling over.

"Now, who did this?" I wanted to know.

The waitress placed the cake in the middle of the table. "Your sons," she told me.

Fred, Paul, and David all looked at each other in bewilderment. "We did not," they said in unison.

Then we all looked at Gary, who was beaming like a searchlight. "I did!" he said proudly.

"Oh, are *you* the young man who called us this afternoon?" the waitress asked. "He called and told us he wanted a cake and some singing. Happy anniversary, Mr. and Mrs. Wallin."

I couldn't get over it. My five-year-old *mizinik,* all by himself, with no prompting, no help, had done this.

"We didn't know a thing about it," Fred assured me.

I think they were all proud of him that night. When we got home, they really gave him the royal treatment.

"So why are you being so nice to me?" Gary chided them with a twinkle in his black cherry eyes. "'Cause we got a big chocolate cake in the refrigerator or something?"

They got along great most of the time, my kids, but of course they fought from time to time as brothers will and got rough with each other.

One evening while I was in the kitchen preparing chopped liver for dinner, Jack's favorite dish, I heard a tremendous crash in the living room and ran in to see what it was all about.

Paul and David were standing over Gary, who was writhing on the floor with his arms locked over his head.

"What happened?" I yelled, bending over Gary and trying to straighten him out.

"We just fell on him and his arms got stuck," Paul said, in awe of the weird position Gary was in.

Gary was screaming and carrying on, but finally we stood him up, walked him around with his arms over his head, and tried to assure him that he was going to be okay.

I called our family doctor, Dr. Eisen, and he told me to get Gary to the emergency room as soon as I could. We took Gary, arms overhead, to the closest hospital, where he promptly received over twenty x-rays. I noticed that his body wasn't covered with a lead shield. I didn't like the idea of Gary's little body absorbing all those deadly rays, and yet I stood in the doorway watching and said nothing.

Not a word. I tried to tell myself the doctors knew what they were doing. And with all those x-rays, they still couldn't relocate Gary's arms.

Later that evening, I kept bugging Jack with questions. "Why did the doctors have to give Gary so many x-rays? Didn't they know that x-rays can cause cancer? Why didn't the doctors use the proper protection? Do you think they could be harmful to Gary?"

"Of course they're not going to be harmful. Would doctors do something that was going to hurt the kid?" Jack answered.

But I was worried. I'd been reading about the dangers of x-rays for years. I knew that any amount of exposure to diagnostic x-rays carries with it a small but a real risk. Every time x-rays pass through living cells, an occasional cell becomes damaged. And the effects are cumulative. So what good was all my reading if I didn't know how to apply it in real life?

The next day I took Gary to an orthopedic doctor and let them take x-rays again. This time the doctor managed to unlock Gary's arms.

Gary never held a grudge after a fight, though at times I think he resented being the youngest. His temper flared when he was left out of things because of his age.

One night we had a *bar mitzvah* to go to and we couldn't take Gary because he had a bad cold. I asked Mama to stay with Gary and he was mad as hell about that, because his brothers were all going, and he was going to be left out.

It was the usual affair in a synagogue in Beverly Hills. One of my friends' sons had come of age, and she made it a lavish occasion—everyone decked out in evening clothes, an orchestra, dancing, and plenty of food. But my heart wasn't in the celebration because I knew how Gary felt about being left at home.

During the festivities I called Mama to check on Gary. She told me Gary had not stopped crying since we left.

I gathered the family and raced home. When I walked

to his room, he was sobbing into his pillow. I sat down on his bed. "Okay, *mizinik,*" I said. "What's all the crying about?"

He wouldn't answer, so I turned him over and brushed the tears from his flushed face. I held him in my arms and explained that I'd only left him home because he wasn't feeling well.

He just kept bawling, so I walked him into the bathroom, washed his face, and then took him back to my bedroom. I rocked him in my rocking chair, singing softly, spoiling him rotten I guess, but so what? I would rather have been in that rocking chair with him than any place else on earth. His head was feverish and he was all stopped up from the cold and crying.

I was a little worried about Gary. He'd been getting sick a lot. Colds off and on every other day, fevers, chills, no appetite.

Finally he fell asleep and I carried him into his room. I tucked him into bed and placed a hand on his hot little forehead.

He'd be all right, I told myself. He'd be fine.

I made sure the other boys were in bed, said goodnight to Mama, and then climbed wearily into bed. I decided to keep Gary home from school the next day and make an appointment with Dr. Eisen.

Maybe, I thought, it was just an allergy.

# Chapter 3

**B**Y THE SPRING OF 1964 I was beginning to fear that there was something seriously wrong with Gary. He'd had frequent colds since he was four years old, but at first that didn't worry me much. Both Dr. Eisen and Gary's pediatrician told me the colds were nothing to worry about, that Gary would outgrow them. They prescribed antibiotics and dismissed us. So Gary was constantly on medication, and I kept waiting for him to outgrow his colds.

By the time he was six, the colds were becoming more frequent instead of less. They came and went from day to day and were usually accompanied by slight fevers.

He didn't seem to have any appetite, either, which worried me. How was he going to get well if he wouldn't eat? My kid was scrawny, and that's an insult to a Jewish mother. Not that she wants her kid fat, just healthy looking. Gary did not look healthy.

I tried to make him eat—tried bribing him, scolding

him, punishing him, pleading with him. But he just wasn't hungry. Of course he never passed up a cream-filled cupcake or a bag of potato chips, so I figured maybe he was just a normal kid. I fed my kids junk food just like most mothers in my generation. We weren't as aware in those days of the dangers of such foods.

When the black and blue marks started appearing all over Gary's body, I began to get even more suspicious that something might be seriously wrong with him. As a medical typist I'd read about leukemia, and, of course, the cases interested me, since they usually involved children. I knew that leukemic children hemorrhage under the skin.

The fear remained undefined in the back of my mind, but I grew increasingly concerned when I examined Gary's bruises, probing around the discolored areas. It was the year that President Kennedy's physical fitness programs were being implemented in the public schools, and I told myself that maybe the increased activity was causing the bruises.

I was relieved when our pediatrician finally suggested that we take Gary in for a tonsillectomy to clear up the incessant colds. He was admitted to the hospital, but after a blood count was taken, the doctor told me that he would not be able to perform the surgery, because Gary was anemic.

Again I was told not to worry. They gave me some pills and I just kept popping them down Gary's throat.

When my son Paul was found to be an anemic infant, I put him on a special diet: raw liver, raw fruits and vegetables, nothing canned, fresh vegetable and fruit juices and vitamins. Eventually Paul's anemia went away.

I wish I had put Gary on that diet. But I just figured the pills were going to take care of it. It was, after all, the age of the magic pill.

But the magic pills didn't seem to work. And he began to complain all the time that his stomach hurt. I took him to the doctors for his stomachaches, and all the doctors could tell me was "Indigestion" or "Nerves" or "Touch of the flu."

I couldn't seem to build up Gary's blood count, and he had another of his bad colds the day before Halloween. This time when the doctor examined him, feeling his abdomen, he told me Gary's liver and spleen were enlarged and that I should take him to the Children's Hospital immediately.

"What could it be, doctor?" I wanted to know. "Is it serious?"

"Probably not at all," the doctor told me. "Could be mononucleosis or maybe cat fever. You have a cat?"

I nodded.

"Well, sometimes a nip from a cat can produce cat fever and that could be all this is. But you take him on over to the Children's Hospital and let them examine him, and they'll be able to treat it for you, whatever it is."

It was chilly the morning we walked through the swinging doors of the Children's Hospital, Gary's hand in mine, our fingers linked. His hands were cold and sweaty. And so frail.

I hated taking him to the hospital that day. It was Halloween and he had wanted to go trick or treating with his brothers. I kept telling him and myself that of course he would go trick or treating. As soon as he was tested, we'd be on our way, costumed, with trick or treat bag in hand.

I checked him in, got him into his pajamas, and we read together most of the day. We read pages alternately, as we did at home.

"In the evening, the boys were shown to their bedrooms," I read. "They climbed into bed quickly, but alas, Eddie the Elephant and Hilda the Hippo were too big to fit into them. So the king ordered the swimming pool emptied and filled with pillows."

I rubbed Gary's neck as I did at home when we were reading together and continued to read. "'And I am so very sleepy,' Eddie sighed. 'A swimming place is a very comfortable place.'"

Gary yawned. "Makes me sleepy reading this," he said with a grin. "Mommy, why am I so sleepy in the middle of the day?"

Before I could answer, I felt three almond-shaped nodes swimming on the back of Gary's neck. Chills and nausea enveloped me. Nodes—they were another symptom of leukemia.

I felt like throwing up. I knew what the doctors were going to tell me. And yet how could I allow such thoughts? How could I be so negative in my thinking?

The determining factor in leukemia is a bone marrow test, a stubby needle plunged through the skin and into the breastbone in order to withdraw cells from the blood factory of the bone marrow, because the marrow is the key to diagnosis and treatment.

When the doctor told me he wanted to perform a bone marrow test on Gary, I tried to forget all the books or magazine articles or watching of the television medical programs which spelled out in plain words what a doctor was looking for when he ordered a test like that.

That evening Gary went in for a bone marrow test and Jack and I waited until midnight for the results. Jack had managed to be there that night—one of the rare occasions in all Gary's sickness. The tests were painful. We heard Gary cry in the treatment room. I wanted to flee, to run out of the hospital doors with my hands over my ears. I didn't want to hear any of it. And I didn't want to hear what the doctors had to say, either.

But at twelve we knew. The doctors told us Gary had acute lymphatic leukemia—cancer of the blood-forming organs. And even though I'd half expected the diagnosis, I was entirely shocked by the words: "I'm sorry, Mr. and Mrs. Wallin, but Gary has acute lymphatic leukemia."

Then they told us about their miracle drugs, the medicine that wouldn't quite cure him, just prolong his life.

"No longer than a year," they said. "Take Gary around the world on a cruise."

I stood there limply, though my body felt as if someone had just thrown a bucket of ice water over me. I wanted to scream, and the kind of mother I was, it wouldn't have been out of character, I guess. Had I started pulling my hair, beating my chest, and gnashing my teeth, it would have been just like me. Overemotional and overwrought. I just wasn't the calm, cool, collected type. But that night, for some odd reason, I was. It was as if someone or something had taken charge of my faculties and had me under control. Controlled but incredulous.

And talk about control. Jack. Jack acted as if someone had just told him Gary had a mild infection. I asked him if he was okay.

"I'm okay," he said. "How about you?"

"Jack," I gasped, "Gary has leukemia. Leukemia, Jack. That means he might die."

I think he just shrugged. Actually I didn't see him shrug, but that was always his attitude. "Oh well, such is life. You win some. You lose some." Just like his gambling.

Dear God, I thought, couldn't the possibility of Gary's dying affect Jack? So what if he'd seen some of his buddies shot down in action during World War II. This was his son.

Jack never took a stand on anything. Life happened to him. He never made things happen. We had come from different places. I was raised so that *nothing* in life *happened* to me. My father taught me to be an *actor*, not a *reactor*. With Jack, it was just the opposite. The thought that life could be controlled never occurred to him. I'm sure it must have saved him a lot of pain. He could let anything roll off him by simply saying, "That's life."

I knew he loved Gary. He loved all his sons. I knew he had emotions. But I wanted to see them. I wanted to see him tremble, suffer, agonize. I wanted proof that he felt something.

I wanted to say something terribly cruel to Jack that night when the doctor told us Gary had leukemia. I wanted to say, "Now it doesn't matter that you wouldn't be an Indian Guide with Gary." Maybe if I had said something like that, it would have evoked a response in Jack. Even anger would have been better than his godawful stillness, his empty quietness.

Jack and I walked back to see Gary. The small hospital room was dark except for the night light by the door, which cast soft shadows against the wall. Gary was fast asleep, his eyelashes stuck to his cheek from crying. His favorite toy was a stuffed pink poodle and he was holding it pressed to his face. The Elvis Presley record he had brought had dropped to the floor. He looked so beautiful. How could he be so deathly ill? My heart wrenched as I watched his breathing, the slow motion of his body. "Gary, my darling *mizinik,*" I whispered softly, "I love you so much. So much. Please don't die. Please."

That night I dreamed that I was running endlessly trying to catch up with Gary to give him the one pill in the world that would make him well. Yet, even as I ran, I knew there was no such pill, no such hope, and that it was all just a dream.

The next morning, Sunday, November 1, at 11 A.M., Jack and I picked Gary up from the Children's Hospital. He was packed and waiting for us. He was standing at the nurse's stand, talking and laughing with one of the nurses. I called "Gary" and he ran to me and hugged me and put his arms tightly around my neck and I glanced up and met the nurse's eyes. Her look told me all that there was in store for Gary, all the torture he would have to endure.

Gary was so glad to be going home that he went skipping down the hall, clutching a coloring book in his hand. It was hard to keep up with him. I was walking along as though it were any other day, as if he had a cold or something and I had an antibiotic in my purse that I was going to give him when we got home.

What was the matter with me that I wasn't shrieking or throwing myself on the floor? I was a chicken-soup mother, wasn't I? A mother who went out of her mind if one of her kids hit his head on a door. And in my purse I was carrying a small bottle of Prednisone, the first of the four drugs that Gary was to take that could prolong his life. If Gary were lucky and managed to achieve a remission, he could live a year at the most. If not, he would be dead within a few months.

With leukemia, Gary had a time-bomb inside him. We didn't know when it would go off during that year, but we knew for sure it would. All the drugs could do was give him time. That was what was in store for Gary. He was doomed the day he was diagnosed—as assuredly as Edmond O'Brien was dead in the movie *D.O.A.* We just had to wait for the bomb to go off.

When we picked up Gary that Sunday morning, I had been able to listen when the doctor started to explain about leukemia. The only way to do anything for Gary was to try to understand what was happening to him, no matter how I felt, and so I listened carefully.

Leukemia, the doctor said, is cancer of the tissues that manufacture blood cells. The tissues are the bone marrow and the lymph glands. Leukemic cells, produced in abundance by the bone marrow, are immature and useless. They actually become predators in the blood, attacking the body's main organs and blocking out the healthy cells.

Leukemic victims usually die of infection because the blood is so deprived of normal blood cells that the immune process is atrophied to the point of nonexistence. Further complications include the massing of the deadly cells, which causes blood vessel deterioration and leads to uncontrollable bleeding.

Ordinarily one of the missions of the white blood cells produced by the bone marrow is to fight infection and disease. Healthy white blood cells produce antibodies which seek out and destroy viruses, bacteria, and debris. In leukemia, the white cells are sick, crazy, and instead of maturing to the point of performing these vital defensive duties, they turn on the body itself, spreading wildly, invading healthy tissue, breaking it down and raging on to total destruction.

In the week that followed, I learned from the doctors at the Children's Hospital that there were only four drugs used to prolong the life of leukemic victims: Prednisone, 6-Mercaptopurine, Methotrexate, and Vincristine. And that's all those drugs could do—prolong life—not save it.

As far as I was concerned, that was impossible. Gary wasn't going to die. Why should he? He had as much right to live as any other kid. He hadn't done anything wrong. Why should he die? Someone was going to save his life. I was going to see to it.

I asked the doctors at the Children's Hospital what other treatments were being tried. What kinds of experiments were going on? Surely someone was trying to save the lives of leukemic victims.

No. All they could offer were these four drugs. He would take them in progression. As he went steadily downhill, he would go on to the next drug. Until there were no more drugs to take.

So I started looking around for doctors. Good ones. The best. I was going to get Gary the best doctor I could find and my kid was going to be okay.

I also started reading a lot. Leukemia was suddenly the most engrossing, important subject in the world. I picked up every magazine, medical journal, newspaper, and book I could find on leukemia. I left my house and the boys to Mama and spent nearly all of my time at the UCLA biomedical library doing my own research.

My reading pointed to the fact that there were indeed other methods of treatment. I didn't have to pump four life-prolonging drugs into Gary and watch him die eventually. Evidently, people were interested in saving lives, and they were experimenting.

The first thing I seized upon was bone marrow transplants. Dr. George Mathe was experimenting with these transplants in France, and there seemed to be a lot of research in that area. They gave a dose of cobalt radiation lethal enough to kill the malignant bone marrow cells in the patient, and then an injection of healthy bone marrow into the bloodstream.

But it was a very experimental treatment. Hardly anyone was really doing it in the United States. Most experiments were taking place in other countries.

I found a hematologist in Beverly Hills who knew what I was talking about when I mentioned bone marrow transplants, and not only that, he agreed that some of the results with the treatment seemed promising. He actually held out some hope that with such treatment Gary might live. If nothing else, maybe he would live longer.

So that settled it. Dr. Hemp would be Gary's doctor. We started visiting him regularly. Dr. Hemp kept Gary on Prednisone, the same drug Children's Hospital had prescribed. It was a tiny white pill that Gary was to take sixteen times a day. The doctor said a bone marrow transplant would come later, after the drug took effect.

That was in November, and by late December, Gary was better. After another painful bone marrow test, the doctor walked Gary out to me in the waiting room and said, "Here's your Chanukah present, Bernice."

The test had shown that Gary's white blood count was down. An overproduction of white blood cells in the bone marrow is characteristic of leukemia. Gary was in remission! If a blood count were taken at this point, no one could detect that Gary had leukemia.

It was a glorious present. Gary seemed to be feeling better. He looked better. The fever was gone. The nodes were gone, and I began to entertain the foolish notion that maybe Gary was going to beat the disease.

I took that opportunity to try to make the family close again. I had been spending so much time with doctors, at libraries, and with Gary, that my other three sons hardly knew me any more.

I had a big Chanukah party to celebrate Gary's remission. Of course I never told anyone that's what we were celebrating. Only Fred, Jack, and I knew.

I never told Paul or David and I never told Gary he was terminally ill. Only Fred. Fred and I didn't talk about it much, but it was a comfort to me, knowing someone else shared my burden. Fred became very solemn in those days, and especially devoted to his little brother. I needed that more than anything else.

The Chanukah party was a festive affair. I had tons and tons of food and lots of family and friends at the house. I pretended everything was normal. Everything was fine.

But I wasn't ignorant. I knew it was just a remission. And I knew remissions didn't last.

Soon Gary started having pain again. Chills, fevers, and frequent nosebleeds. He had to be rushed to the hospital to get his nose packed and to get transfusions. He couldn't eat.

"But Mommy, I have a stomachache," he would groan at the table. "Do I have to eat?"

"You have to, Gary," I told him firmly.

But he would gag on his food, throw up after a few mouthfuls, and I knew leukemic cells had returned.

I asked Dr. Hemp when we would begin the bone marrow transplant. He said it might not be called for in Gary's case.

"What do you mean, not called for?" I demanded. "What does it take to be called for?"

"Mrs. Wallin, you'll have to trust my judgment in these things. I'm a specialist. I know all about Gary's disease. And I will know when it's time to try something different."

By that time I wasn't sure I trusted him. What was it Papa had said about doctors? "A *mench vee alleh menchen.*"

I continued to read. And I read about a doctor named

Celia Rosenfeld who was doing an experimental treatment on leukemic patients. She isolated the cancerous cells from the urine and made a vaccine. An autogenous vaccine, she called it. The vaccine was supposed to build up the immune defenses, and these defenses were supposed to fight leukemia.

I took Gary to see her. We tried the therapy, and for a while it seemed to work. For two months he seemed to improve.

But it was only for two months. And then came the heavy nosebleeds again. Again we had to rush him to the hospital for transfusions and medication.

One of the customers from the butcher shop where Jack worked called me one day and mentioned that she had read an interesting article written by a well-known hematologist in Boston, Massachusetts, but that she had inadvertently thrown out the magazine. She said this doctor seemed to think he had some answers. She gave me the doctor's name so that I could locate the article.

I went to a couple of libraries but couldn't locate the article. So I tried calling Information in Boston to see if they had a listing for Dr. William Dameshek. They did.

I called Dr. Dameshek and we discussed Gary's illness. When I asked him what he thought caused leukemia, he said, "I am convinced, Mrs. Wallin, that leukemia is the result of an impaired, altered, or abnormal immune system." He wasn't like the other doctors I had spoken with. He had an air of confidence. He sounded so sure about what he was saying.

I told him that the treatments Gary had gotten from Dr. Rosenfeld supposed to have had something to do with the immune system, and I asked him what he thought. He believed Dr. Rosenfeld's treatments were based on sound medical practice, but he pointed out to me what I already knew so well, that by the time leukemia is diagnosed, it is already so far disseminated throughout the body that it is impossible to arrest.

I went back to Dr. Hemp and demanded that we start the bone marrow transplant immediately.

Again he hedged. "All the factors have to be weighed carefully, Bernice," he said. "As you well know, this treatment is highly experimental. We can't just . . ."

"Yes, I know they're experimental, Dr. Hemp. But so what?" I replied. "When we talked about it last year they were experimental. That didn't seem to bother you then. So now what's the problem? If I'm willing to try it, why shouldn't you be?"

"First of all, the donor has to be exactly matched to the patient. And it's not always easy to find a willing donor with an exact match."

"Well what about me? Or one of my sons? Wouldn't one of my family be likely to have an exact match? Come on, Dr. Hemp, we have to try it."

We got as far as testing the three boys, and we found that Fred had the match needed for a transplant. My hopes went up a little.

Still Dr. Hemp hesitated. "Let's wait a while," he said.

I told him I was fed up with the waiting. I asked him what he knew about another treatment I'd read about— cellular therapy it was called. They were doing it in other countries, such as Switzerland and Germany, but not in the United States.

"That's just another one of those way-out treatments, Bernice. You're grasping at straws, and I think if we start playing around like that, we're likely to lose ground."

"Likely? We've already lost ground!" I screamed at him. "6-MP was too toxic for his system and this third drug, Methotrexate, you've got him on doesn't seem to be doing him any good. We've waited and waited, Dr. Hemp. Don't you see it could be too late?"

I investigated the cellular therapy theory and found that some doctors were holding out some real hope with these treatments. It involved the injecting of an extract from the placentae of freshly slaughtered lambs into cancer patients, where the sick cells could possibly be stimulated by the healthy cells to produce antibodies. It also had something to do with building up the immune system, I thought.

It sounded gross. It sounded like a quack cure, I admitted to myself. But I reasoned that down through the ages, new concepts in medicine had sometimes sounded crazy and had often been met with opposition and scorn. In time some of these concepts were found to be perfectly correct and sound.

I called the Paul Neihans Clinic in Montreux Clairens, Switzerland, where they were giving cellular therapy, and talked with a doctor there who spoke English. We discussed the treatment they were giving at the clinic. He recommended that I take Gary to Tijuana right away, the nearest place he could receive the cellular therapy.

He went on to say that people were getting good results from this therapy. Hope began to surface.

I went to Dr. Hemp and told him I'd decided to take Gary to Tijuana for treatments.

"You're crazy," he told me.

"Why? Why am I crazy? Because I want to try to save my child's life? All you want to do is watch him die, doctor. That's the feeling I get, because you are offering me nothing. Absolutely nothing!"

"Mrs. Wallin, I highly resent that statement. I am a respected physician who has the well-being of his patients in mind. Now if you want to truck off to Tijuana for some quack treatment, that is your business. I, as a professional, am telling you that it is not going to help."

I started to cry. "But Dr. Hemp, there are other doctors who say they've tried these treatments and seen good results. Couldn't you just look into it? Couldn't you just consult with one of these doctors for the sake of my son? What if it did help?"

"I will not consult with these doctors in Tijuana, Bernice. That's final. It would be going against my better judgment. And I never do that."

"Then I won't be seeing you again, Dr. Hemp," I said. "I'm taking Gary out of your care."

Crying, I left his office and made arrangements to get Gary into the clinic in Tijuana. At that point, quackery was better than what Dr. Hemp was doing, which, as far as I was concerned, was simply pill-pushing.

I wanted desperately to sit down with Jack and discuss Gary's illness. I wanted to ask him if I was doing the right thing for Gary by switching to the treatments in Tijuana. And I tried. His replies were, "How should I know what's right," "Don't ask me what to do," and "Do what you want to do."

"Who is going to help me if you can't?" I screamed at him.

So I had to make the decision myself.

# Chapter 4

On the morning of my first trip to Tijuana with Gary, I was combing my hair in front of the bathroom mirror when I realized how haggard I was beginning to look. I was thirty-eight years old and I looked fifty. My hair was stringy. My complexion was sallow. There were dark circles under my eyes.

Besides that, I wasn't feeling well. My breasts and shoulders ached. I thought I might be suffering from bursitis or arthritis. Maybe it was stress or exhaustion, I told myself.

There was a suspicious lump in my right breast, which I had anxiously probed that morning. My breasts had been filled with cysts since Gary was born, but this lump was growing.

That morning, however, I didn't have time to think about myself. I threw on a combination of clothing, which hung limply on my skinny body. I looked like a tramp. But the least of my worries was how I looked.

The three boys were going with us to Tijuana since Mama wasn't feeling well and I thought it might be good company for Gary to have his brothers along. The thought of making that long trip frightened me. I hated freeway driving. But I had no choice. I knew Jack would never ask his boss for time off from work.

The boys played rather hysterically that morning. They had all been a little hyperactive since Gary's illness had set in, especially Gary. The painful treatments and the constant blood counts were nerve-wracking for him, and he became almost devilish in his play.

The kids argued a lot while I was getting ready. Gary got mad at one of his brothers and ran outside, slamming the door behind him.

When it was time to leave, I found him in the back yard bending over his vegetable garden, staring lovingly at some of the green shoots that were pushing their way through the earth. I caressed the back of his feverish neck.

"Look, Mommy, the corn's starting to come up," he said with wonder. "And look over there. Are those the tomatoes?"

"Yup," I said. "They're going to be big, too, I bet. Big, red juicy tomatoes, Gary."

"Yuck. Too bad I hate tomatoes."

"You don't hate tomatoes, Gary," I said. "You've always loved tomatoes. Chilled right out of the refrigerator, sliced, with salt and pepper. Remember?"

He stood up weakly and put his hands on his hips. "I don't like them any more," he said sadly. He looked up at me and it almost made me sick to see the yellow tinge in his skin. "Mommy, when am I going to be over this anemia?"

I hugged him. We embraced a minute, the warm sun on our backs, his thin little arms around my waist. "Pretty soon, honey," I told him. "Pretty soon. And you'll be able to eat the corn and the tomatoes and some of those carrots we planted and everything else. That's why we're taking you to Tijuana today. The doctors have a new treatment they think is going to make you well real quick."

He tightened his grip around my waist. "Is it going to hurt? Like at Dr. Hemp's? Is it going to hurt bad like that?"

I sighed and bit my lip. "I don't know, honey. We'll just have to wait and see. But you know, Gary, I wouldn't let anyone hurt you for anything, unless I thought it was going to make you all better real soon. You know that, don't you?"

He let go of my waist, looked back at his vegetable garden and said, "Yeah, I know that. You love me. I know." Then he glanced up at me and I saw a shadow of that familiar impish grin of his. "I love you, too," he said. "Let's go."

There was an almost endless stream of cars and trucks all the way from Los Angeles to San Diego. By the time we crossed the Mexican border, I was a nervous wreck. Gary lay sprawled across the back seat, oblivious to the yelling and giggling of his brothers. Too exhausted to join in. Too sick to sleep.

Baja, California, was anything but a reassuring place to be taking Gary for treatment. Tijuana is a massive slum, but it was also my last hope. The clinic was not exactly spic and span. I almost turned around and left when I saw the dingy, dirty carpet, the worn furniture, the filthy walls and general disarray.

The place was mobbed with Americans, all of them milling around, talking with one another as if it were any other kind of clinic, and not a clinic of last resort. I had expected to see a depressing bunch of deathly-ill people, moaning and writhing and carrying on, but instead they were friendly people, people who wanted to talk about their illness and the treatment they were on. And I talked with dozens of them that day.

One woman, beautiful and young, the wife of a U.S. senator, introduced herself and told me the American medical system had given up on her. She was suffering from a type of bone-marrow cancer, myeloma. She told me that after three months of Laetrile treatments, she was feeling stronger and had no pain whatever.

I'd heard a little about Laetrile, but it was long before all the controversy over it. There had been scattered articles published on some of its favorable results. I knew it had something to do with a vitamin, but I didn't know how it worked.

"Well, it all started with a man named Dr. Krebs," she explained. "He started working with Laetrile several years ago and from his experiments he advanced the theory that cancer is a deficiency disease aggravated by the lack of an essential compound in modern man's diet. And he feels that the ultimate control of cancer is to be found simply in restoring this substance—I think it's called 'nitriloside'— anyway, he named it 'vitamin B17.' It's found in natural foods we don't get much of these days. Like apricot seeds, millet, bitter almonds. What else? Apple seeds. Things we just don't eat anymore. But that's what Laetrile is. A concentration of this substance, this B17 we've been lacking in our diets."

I shook my head skeptically. "Sounds pretty oversimplified to me," I said.

"I know it does, Bernice, but I believe in Laetrile. And I'll bet every single person you talk to here also believes in it."

She was right. They all did believe in it. Some of them had come in dying. Some of them were dragged in by their family and friends. And almost all of them had the same story to tell. American doctors had told them to go home and die, that there was no hope. But after a few months of Laetrile, some of them told me, their appetite was increased, they were gathering strength, even gaining weight. Boy, did my hopes surge.

The wait for Gary's appointment was long, and by the time we got in to see the doctor, it was evening. The kids were going crazy. It was all I could do to keep them from tearing up the reception room.

The doctor who examined Gary was one who had studied under Dr. Paul Niehans in Switzerland. We had spoken on the phone several times before this visit, and he was familiar with Gary's case.

He told me about the treatments Gary was going to get. I was curious about Laetrile. I wanted to know more about it. But the doctor said Gary was there mainly for the cellular therapy, though he would be taking Laetrile as supplemental treatment.

After we'd discussed Gary's history at length, he examined Gary and gave him five or six injections. By now, Gary was used to the battery of needles always shooting into his tender skin. He held my hand and gritted his teeth.

Included in the treatment were blood cleansing shots which the doctor said came from Germany. He gave me a strict diet for Gary to follow. No white sugar or flour, no foods with preservatives or additives, no carbonated drinks, no meat. Only raw fruits and vegetables, whole grains and fish. The doctor explained that the chemistry of the body can sometimes be altered through proper nutrition, so as to eliminate disease. It sounded sensible to me. Everyone knows that diet can influence a person's health in a remarkable way. And, anyway, wasn't it Hippocrates who, twenty-five hundred years ago, said, "Let thy food be thy medicine and let thy medicine be thy food"?

It was nine o'clock before we were on our way home. I drove back into the United States reassured. The doctor had offered no false hopes. But he hadn't called Gary's case a hopeless one either. I liked that. I also realized that as a desperate mother fighting for her son's life, I was likely to be taken in by anything that sounded hopeful. But at that point I decided that one major qualifying factor in choosing a doctor was to find one who didn't give up hope. One who was willing to try anything and everything.

But how ironic, I thought as I drove back with a car full of sleeping children, back to the land of plenty, to the land where freedom reigns. Why in the hell did I have to drive to another country for hope? It was ridiculous.

I took Gary to the clinic in Tijuana two or three times a week for treatments. But after two months he was still fading. We tried more concentrated doses of Laetrile, in addition to all the other medications and treatments he was getting, but nothing seemed to help. I couldn't give up, though. It was the only treatment that offered any hope.

It was sometime during the third or fourth month of Gary's treatments in Tijuana that I had an accident. I was particularly worn out that day and the unusually hot weather didn't help any.

I had been up since five that morning packing a styrofoam ice chest with the food that Gary was allowed to eat. The freeway had been jammed and I had barely escaped getting sideswiped.

With Gary holding my hand, we crossed the crowded Tijuana street and headed for the doctor's office. Parked in front of the medical building was a donkey-drawn cart overflowing with fresh fruit, vegetables, and juices.

I asked Gary if he'd like something cool to drink and he nodded his head yes. As we neared the cart, I stepped off the curb to approach the vendor. Slam! I don't know what I slipped on but I fell flat on my face. Blook spurted from my nose and lips and all I saw was red. Then the pain! I felt two strong hands under my armpits and the next thing I knew, I was on my feet. I reached out and felt my nose. Blood oozed through my fingers and down the front of my blouse. I looked up at Gary and he was screaming. I tried to tell him that I was okay.

I heard a voice offer me a handkerchief and I put it up to my face. I pointed toward the medical building and somehow the man understood my garbled speech and helped Gary and me up the stairs to the doctor's office. Gary thanked him.

At the doctor's appointment, I was the first to get examined. After they cleaned up the blood, the doctors were able to determine my nose was broken in three places. Sitting in the waiting room with an ice pack on my nose while Gary got his treatment, I took a mirror out of my purse and looked at myself. My God, I was a sorry sight. What used to be a small, short, nice nose was now smashed flat across my face and looked ugly.

I pushed the mirror back into my purse, as tears started to fill my eyes. What's to be excited about, I thought? For a broken nose there's always a Beverly Hills plastic surgeon. For Gary—who knows?

In all those trips back and forth to Tijuana I was in constant fear that one day my aging automobile would break down in the middle of Mexico. I didn't know a word of Spanish and I was afraid we might be stuck for days.

One day my fear was realized. The car broke down about twenty miles from the clinic. I had been watching the temperature gauge and it was registering hot by the time we crossed the border. The car began to make a squealing sound and smoke poured from under the hood. I got out of the car, dragging Gary with me, and we watched it hiss and sizzle.

Gary was doubled over, holding his stomach and groaning. I laid him down by the side of the road, propping his head on my jacket. I was panic-stricken. Now what?

Fortunately, a nice man from Los Angeles stopped his car and asked if he could help us. I explained, making certain that Gary couldn't hear me, that I was just on my way to the clinic with a son dying of leukemia. The man raced off to the nearest phone and called the police.

The police arrived promptly, sirens screaming. They listened to my story and called a tow truck from their car. There was nothing they could do to repair the car, so I asked them to tow it into Los Angeles. They told me it would have to be towed to Tijuana, where it would remain until I picked it up. I watched as it was lifted and towed away, not knowing if I'd ever see the old jalopy again.

The police drove us to the clinic. They spoke a little English and tried to make small talk with me, though it was difficult with Gary moaning in the back seat next to me. Occasionally they'd glance back over their shoulders with looks of concern and sympathy.

After Gary's treatment at the clinic, we took a taxi back to the border, walked across, and boarded a bus headed for San Diego. From there we got on a train and I rode back to Los Angeles with Gary lying in my lap, our supply of Laetrile tucked into the wig I had purchased specifically to conceal the illegal drug. It was especially harrowing that day, because the Laetrile had to be smuggled across the border. I always hid it in my underwear or under the dashboard of the car, and no one had ever asked to search us. When we went over the border, the immigration officials always saw Gary lying pitifully on the back seat and waved us through immediately. But that day, what with the taxis and walking over the border and the trains and all the confusion, I was terrified that we'd be caught and sent to jail.

We made it home, though. Jack picked me up at the train station and I made arrangements for picking up the car on our next visit.

All the time I was taking Gary to Mexico, I was also having Gary's blood tested in Los Angeles to be sure that it showed the same results that the doctor in Tijuana claimed. I wasn't being deceived. The blood test results were the same.

Finally the doctors in Tijuana told me to take Gary home and put him in a hospital. There was nothing else they could do for him, they said. And when they, my last hope, they who had seemed to have hope themselves, when they told me he had only a few weeks to live, I was broken.

I hadn't been able to get the doctors in the United States

to do a bone marrow transplant, and all of my feverish research had led to nothing more than a huge medical bill in Tijuana. Gary had been doomed from the start and nothing I had done or tried to do had made a bit of difference. I was bitter against everyone.

Whether Laetrile or cellular therapy worked or not would never be proven by Gary. It was too late.

The day they gave me the news, I drove back over the border and stopped at the first pay phone I could find to call Dr. Hemp. I asked him if he would take Gary back under his care.

"Of course I'll take him back, Bernice. Did they take him off the drugs while you were down in Tijuana?" he yelled at me over the phone. "You took him to a bunch of quacks."

"Please, doctor, don't yell at me. I had to try. I just had to. Everyone said he would die, and no one was willing to try anything different."

"Then get him back to me as soon as you possibly can. He never should have been off those drugs for one minute."

Gary was asleep beside me on the front seat of the car as we drove home. His breathing was labored and irregular.

My mind was racing like the fast cars that were passing me by on the freeway. Did I think that somehow I had the power to do for Gary what the doctors couldn't? Was I playing God? Had I shortened Gary's life by taking him off the drugs? Had I shortened his life even for a moment?

The trip back to Culver City was filled with silent madness as I cried quietly, squeezing the steering wheel in a stranglehold that was meant for everybody who had failed my son, including myself.

Dr. Hemp met me at the back entrance of a hospital in Culver City. Gary had to be carried in on a stretcher because he was doubled up with pain and burning up with fever.

The doctor put Gary on the last drug, Vincristine. But it

was useless. Transfusion after transfusion failed to help, and Gary's grip on life slipped away. His temperature was over 107 degrees and while we packed his feverish body in ice, Gary screamed over and over for me to take him home. "Mommy, I feel like I'm in the twilight zone. Take me home. Please take me home. I'm afraid."

I knew that Gary was talking about "Twilight Zone," Rod Serling's television show, and that he had to be in something very close to the hell I'd heard so much about.

For a few hours, on some of those final days, when Gary's fever dropped a notch or two, we watched television together. We saw Juan Marichal, the San Francisco Giants' pitcher, take the law into his own hands and hit Dodger catcher, John Roseboro, in the head with a bat. Has the whole world gone mad, I thought? The day we saw Watts burning up, I felt as if I was in the twilight zone too. It was August 1965. Mayor Yorty came on the screen and told us all that the National Guard was being sent into the inner city, that the police were going to restore order.

Order? Was there any order to life, I wondered. At that point it would have delighted me if the whole country had burned and we all went up in flames. It would seem fairer somehow. Then Gary wouldn't be alone.

Some of the nurses on the floor were extremely compassionate, especially one named Jean Williams. She watched over Gary devotedly and tried hard to comfort me. She was young and vibrant and healthy-looking, and Gary seemed to respond to her warmth with as much enthusiasm as he could muster.

Fred stayed with me at the hospital during the last week, leaving only when errands had to be run or to bring me a clean change of clothes. His eyes showed the strain he was under. He couldn't stand to be left in the room with the little brother he loved so dearly. We tried to comfort each other, though we rarely spoke. A pat on the back or a look straight into the eyes once in a while—

that's how we spoke to each other in Gary's final days.

Someone notified the rabbi who had confirmed Fred and when he came to the hospital to see Gary, all I could say was, "What are you good for? Gary's dying. I don't need your comforting."

"It's not always given to us to understand why terrible things happen to us," he answered. "But you must realize that it is God's will."

"Please. Please. Go away," I begged. "I don't need you to say things like that. Go away, please."

He walked away, shaking his head from side to side.

I wrote Elvis Presley a letter begging him to call or visit Gary. Since Gary idolized him, he would have been thrilled to see him. The letter came back marked, "Address Unknown."

One day I stood at Gary's bedside, examining his sweet baby face, a face that had once been impish and full of mischievous smiles, now drained of that animation and vitality. I watched him lying there as though he were already dead, pale and sallow, motionless, his face turned toward the window, his eyes ringed with circles, expressing his pain. I walked to the window of the hospital and looked down all seven floors, wondering how it would feel to jump. Then I wouldn't have to witness this. I wouldn't have to cope with his pain, hear him moan and scream out. But how selfish of me. What about my other sons? In a way, I think that's the only thing that kept me from leaping right through the glass. After all, who would care for them if I was gone? Certainly not their father.

I walked away from the window and slumped in a chair, my face buried in my hands. Suddenly I heard a terrible commotion from Gary's bed. I turned and saw Gary twitching violently, gaining momentum with each jerk. His arms were snapping at the elbows. His whole body jumped from the bed, destroying the solid ice packs. The tubes tore loose from his flesh and the IV bottles swayed crazily.

I tried to restrain him. "Jean!" I screamed. "Someone! Help!"

When Jean and another nurse came in, I backed away, terrified. Gary's body looked as if it were being hit with volts of electricity. He jerked and convulsed and writhed.

I fainted.

When I woke up, the doctor was there, and Gary was leaning back against the pillows, breathing strangely, short little breaths. His eyes were dulled and distant, his drawn face almost expressionless.

"Why did he do that, Dr. Hemp?" I whispered in horror.

Dr. Hemp took me by the arm and led me out into the hallway. "Gary has about forty-eight hours to live," he said quietly.

I laughed hysterically. A crackling banshee-cry. "Gary is doing a death dance. Gary is doing a *Totentanz*. A *Totentanz*," I kept repeating. Gary had only forty-eight hours to live. Forty-eight hours. Two goddamn days.

"No! No!" I remember my mind screaming and I think I screamed aloud.

"Damn you," I thought. "All of you, go to hell. Get out of my life. Get out of my son's life. Leave me alone. Leave me to die with my son. Please! Gary! Don't wait. Get it over with. Just die. Damn it. Just die, please, so I can die too. Please!" I broke down, blubbering, cursing, pounding my thighs with my fists, trying to find comfort in biting my lower lip, but only managing to draw blood. I remember feeling a very real comfort from the taste of my own blood.

*Totentanz.* A damn death dance. As if my son had just been to hell and performed an ugly dance to initiate his passage within forty-eight hours. I wanted to defy the gods and demons and angels and spirits of all peoples and all religions in a crazed effort to save my son from inevitability. It wasn't just that he must die. We all die. We start dying the moment we are born. But I couldn't accept that Gary must die at seven . . . only seven years old.

"Please don't let him die, doctor. Please! Do something so that he won't die."

But even as I pleaded, I knew that at a certain point in the treatment of leukemia all further moves are blocked. The body is overrun with the bad cells. Because so many white blood cells are present in the bone marrow, there is no room left for the formation of red blood cells and the platelets that are necessary for clotting to occur. Without them, the slightest, smallest nick or scratch may bleed endlessly. Eventually, the blood vessels, weakened by the general disease, rupture and have no means of repairing themselves. The red blood cells, which act as storage containers for oxygen, are too few. Breathing becomes more difficult; parts of the body that need oxygen are starved for it and die, just as a tree dies without water. Even before the whole body dies, the liver, kidney, the retina of the eye, almost any organ may become devastated by lack of air. And all the white cells do no good, because they are sick, crazy, nonfunctioning. Instead of helping to eat up bacteria and other debris, which is their usual task, they simply float around, clogging and choking blood vessels. Transfusions are the usual means of replacing red blood cells and platelets, but too many transfusions further depress the bone marrow and the formation of blood and cut off the one way in which new and somewhat healthy blood cells might be formed. Transfusion reactions at any moment can be lethal and it is impossible to transfuse a person with blood day after day.

Deep in my heart I knew now that Gary was going to die. Nothing could save him. I felt a violent shooting pain in my chest. My knees were threatening to buckle again. Dr. Hemp put his arms around my shoulders and said somberly, "Bernice, I want you to be prepared for Gary's death."

Prepared! No, I wasn't prepared. And believe it or not,

I still hadn't given up. I may have gone a little mad, but I remember having read an article sometime that week about a doctor right in Los Angeles giving Laetrile shots, and the article had been so positive, so hopeful. I made the necessary arrangements by phone.

When I told Dr. Hemp I was leaving with Gary he was furious. Waving his arms and ranting, he called me an imbecile and a fool.

But Gary was moved by ambulance, encased in an oxygen tent, with the tubes and IV still intact, the doctor fuming, people in the hospital staring, nurses shaking their heads as if they thought I was nuts.

We took him to the Parkview Hospital, where in addition to blood transfusions, he got injections of all kinds, blood-cleansing, Laetrile, Prednisone, 6-MP, Methotrexate and Vincristine. But it was useless.

The last forty-eight hours ran together. There was no morning, no afternoon, no day or night.

Gary lay there in his bed, limp and semiconscious, with tubes running in and out of his body. "Mommy, Mommy, help me; please help me!" he whispered hoarsely. His skin was murky yellow and a mass of blue-black welts. Not an inch of his body was untouched. Bruises, four or five inches across, caused by broken capillaries underneath the skin, covered his arms, chest, and legs—the red and purple dots of petechiae. Symptoms of platelet failure were everywhere. I saw blood beginning to ooze out of the corner of Gary's mouth. Appalled, in the midst of all that was going on, all the paraphernalia, the tubes, the catheters, I watched the drops of blood gathering, growing, getting redder and redder, until, like tears, they began sliding down his body, onto the sheet, the pillow, everywhere. I felt as if my own blood were oozing out of me.

Gary's tongue was swollen and bleeding. His gums, his fingers—his nose, and every bodily orifice dripped blood.

"Look Mommy, look. I'm bleeding. Make me stop bleeding," he begged.

Suddenly he opened his eyes with a wide-fixed stare and said, "Mommy, Mommy," and then he closed them again.

The doctor felt Gary's pulse. "Mrs. Wallin . . . " he said softly.

I knew. Gary was dead.

This child with all his curiosity, all his questions, his fish tanks with their filters, his parakeet flying around the house, the kids who congregated in his room, his doctor's kit and the sign on his door—"Back in one hour"—all those things he'd thought about and wondered about . . . they were all wiped out on August 23, 1965, at 9:40 A.M.

The doctor left the room quietly. But the private nurse who had come on duty at seven in the morning walked over to me, a tall, gaunt woman with short, blond, wispy hair.

I didn't want her sympathy. And she wasn't about to give it. What she said was, "Mrs. Wallin, even if I only worked a couple of hours, I have to get paid for a full day."

Sobbing wildly, I screamed, "You bitch," as I pushed her into the hall and locked the door. I went to the sink and wet a washcloth to wipe the dried blood from Gary's lips and body. Then I got into bed with him and cradled him. He was still warm from breathing, his head limp against my chest.

I heard people knocking at the door, but I didn't move. I just rocked my baby. Back and forth. How he had suffered. How he had suffered. Over and over in my mind. The suffering. Why? Why? Why? Papa! Why? Why?

I don't know how they got in or when, but I felt the morticians lift me, supporting me on both sides and dragging me into the hall. I looked back. The nurse was covering Gary's face with a sheet.

My husband was waiting for me. The doctor had telephoned Jack at work and notified him of Gary's death. "You locked the door," Jack said. "We couldn't get in. You locked the door. Why did you do that?"

But there were no words to say and I was dry-eyed because I had cried every tear to my name.

On the way out of the hospital, I called home and told Fred that Gary had died. A nurse handed me Gary's small suitcase, and I clutched it to my breast all the way home.

When we got home, I walked directly to Gary's room, opened the suitcase, took out his toy pink poodle and the Elvis Presley records, and put them back on his dresser. Then I went straight to the cupboard where we kept the liquor. Not that we ever drank at home, but Jack had received hundreds of bottles of booze for Chanukah and Christmas presents from his customers since starting to work at the butcher shop as far back as 1949. I poured myself a few stiff drinks, and the pain in my heart eased a little. I wasn't used to liquor or feeling high. It was a new sensation. It made everything seem hazy and far away.

I stayed bombed as much as possible that day. I thought about the funeral arrangements, but I couldn't bring myself to do anything about them.

Jack's employer Arnie, and his wife, Helen, came over that evening and brought their poodle with them. Paul and David were entranced by the dog, but Fred stayed in his room with the door shut.

Again I thought about the funeral arrangements. We were flat broke. How do you bury a child without money? Nobody does anything for nothing. Even that.

I had never been able to save any money during our marriage. I didn't consider myself extravagant, but because Jack took so much out of his check for gambling, it had been impossible to make ends meet. My working had helped a little, but I had used that money to add on a den and to improve our home. So when Gary got sick, there was no savings account I could draw from. Not that it would have mattered if I had had a savings account, because the bills were more than $10,000 the first four months of Gary's illness.

In my drunken stupor I remembered the Metropolitan

Life Insurance policies I had purchased for the children's education—two or three dollars a month to be paid up by age eighteen, just in time for college. Gary wouldn't be needing his college money.

I went to the telephone and dialed my insurance agent's home.

Not waiting for a hello, I rushed out with, "Mr. Raber, this is Bernice Wallin. Gary died this morning and I need his insurance money to bury him."

"Oh my God. I'm so sorry. I don't know what to say. I'll do what I can to get you the insurance money promptly. But I do need Gary's death certificate before I can start processing the death claim."

"Certificate? Why?"

"Because all insurance companies require proof of death."

"Believe me. He's dead."

"Bernice, it's a necessary procedure and I'm sorry to have to put you through this."

"It's okay, Mr. Raber. Where do I get Gary's death certificate?"

"The mortuary will send you the certificate in a day or two. Mail it to us when you get it. Okay?"

"Okay."

"I'm sorry, Bernice. I don't know what . . ."

"It's okay, Mr. Raber. What's there to say?" I thanked him and hung up.

Jack was sitting slouched in a chair. Arnie was talking to Paul and David.

I turned to Arnie and asked, "Will you lend us the money to bury Gary until his insurance policy money comes through?"

"Sure, Bernice, how much do you want?"

"Wait, I'll find out."

I looked in the phone book for Groman's Mortuary and dialed their number.

"Please, tell me the price of a casket," I asked. "A small

one, just a little over four feet long. The cheapest one."
And then because I couldn't think of putting Gary into the
ground, I added, "And how much is a crypt?"

"I'll have to look it up. Please stay on the line for a
minute."

I poured myself another drink while I waited.

"Four hundred and sixty-five dollars," the man said
when he came back to the phone. "That is, if you pick the
cheapest casket."

"It's a deal," I answered.

"Don't you want to see it before you buy it?"

"No, what for?"

I turned to Arnie and asked, "Will you lend us $465.00
to bury my son?" Every time I said "bury my son" I
was reminding myself that Gary was really dead.

Arnie wrote out a check for $465.00.

That was Monday evening. We had to decide when to
have the funeral. Jack said tomorrow would be too soon
because we'd have to notify people.

"I don't have to notify anybody," I said. "Gary is dead,
so who cares who knows."

Jack said Gary's funeral would be on Wednesday.

The evening before the funeral, I went to Gary's room
and started pulling things out of his drawers and closets for
him to be buried with. He'd wear his favorite brown
corduroys and definitely a tie—that silly tie he was always
wanting to wear. He'd want some of his favorite Elvis
Presley records with him, his Timex, his doctor's kit, what
else?

When my sister Sally came for the things I had for her
to take to the mortuary, she told me I was crazy. "Bossie,
you can't bury a child with all those things," she told me.

"The hell I can't," I slurred back drunkenly.

And it wasn't easy talking the mortuary into it, either.
But I did. "This is highly irregular," they informed me
pompously.

"To hell with 'highly irregular.' A lot of things are

highly irregular. Was it highly irregular for the Egyptians to bury their dead with their possessions thousands of years ago? He's my son you're burying and this is how I want him buried. So do me something."

Gary was buried just as I asked at Beth Olam Cemetery in a crypt on August 25, 1965, at 10:30 in the morning. I wasn't there. I got so drunk I passed out. Deliberately, I suppose it was. So I wouldn't have to see Gary lying in his casket.

At noon on the day of Gary's funeral my insurance agent phoned to tell me that Gary had exactly $465.00 in paid-up premiums. How's that for a coincidence?

When my family returned from the services, I stayed in my room drinking. Jack came into the bedroom and laid the memorial candle on the dresser. He glanced at me briefly and walked out of the room. I sipped and drank and set my glass back on the table and brooded.

I could hear the clatter of dishes, cupboard doors being opened, chairs being moved, and lots of footsteps. I heard chuckles and faint laughter. And I sat there, staring at the opposite wall. And then again, I heard laughter. I listened, too stunned to react emotionally. My skin crawled. People were making light of my son's death. Is that the way you mourn, my friends, my dear friends? Don't you secretly feel grateful that the son you watched being buried today wasn't your own? Is that why you're laughing, from sheer gratefulness? Don't you have any respect for Gary? To hell with all of you. To hell with you all.

With as much dignity as I could muster, I staggered out to the living room and found our dining room table loaded with food: salami, egg salad, corned beef, boiled potatoes, rye bread. People were piling the food onto paper plates and laughing and carrying on as if they were at a party.

I weaved over to the table and yanked the tablecloth. Dishes, silverware, and food tumbled to the floor. Half of the egg salad landed on my foot.

I glared at Jack. I thought I had told him I didn't want a

wake, though he later swore I had never communicated this wish to him. In my state of mind, it was entirely possible. But he should have known I wouldn't want a wake.

I walked past all the staring, embarrassed people into the kitchen and picked up my real friend—another bottle of bourbon. I went right back to my room and left Jack and Mama to clean up the mess and explain to those people that Bernice was not quite herself since Gary died.

Bernice was just feeling the loss.

About a week later when Mr. Raber, the insurance man, came to deliver the check, Jack was in the kitchen having breakfast. Mr. Raber came into the house carrying his briefcase and sat down on the couch.

"I'm sorry, Bernice, to be here under these tragic circumstances. I do need your signature on a few of these forms," he said, opening the briefcase and taking out some of the papers.

I took the pen he handed me and without glancing at the papers, I signed where he indicated. He closed his briefcase, laid the check on the coffee table and immediately rose and headed for the door. It was obvious he felt uncomfortable and wanted to leave in a hurry.

"Bernice, I just don't know what to say. I pay these death claims every so often and I can never get used to it. I hope the Lord gives you the strength to carry on."

The door closed and he was gone.

Jack came out of the kitchen and picked up the check.

"Good," he said, folding it and putting it into his wallet. "I'll give it to Arnie when I go to work tomorrow."

He went to the bedroom to get his jacket. "I'll see you later," he said as he walked out the door.

I looked at my watch. It was 8:30 A.M. The gambling parlors in Gardena would be open in half an hour.

I went over to the sink, opened the cupboard door, and took out an unopened bottle of dark red wine from the middle shelf. My hands trembled as I sat down. Tears blurred my vision. I unscrewed the top of the bottle, poured a drink, and held the glass out in front of me at eye level, my hand shaking. I tried to look through the wine. The wine was the color of Gary's blood that wasn't flowing anymore. I gulped down the first drink. I filled my glass a second time, a third time, a fourth time, and then I lost count. I got up from the chair and lurched drunkenly to my bedroom. I lay down on my bed and started beating the pillows with both my fists until I must have passed out.

# Chapter 5

I GUESS I DRANK EVERY DAY for about a year after Gary's death. And I didn't drink in moderation either. I got bombed every day.

It didn't make it easier on the family, but for once I wasn't thinking about the family. All I could think about was that Gary was dead. The drinking didn't make me forget that Gary was locked in a crypt forever. It just helped ease the pain, which manifested itself as a deep ache in the center of my chest. The pain seemed to drain all my strength, and often I drank until I passed out or fell asleep. Drunk and asleep, I was safe. Awake, I blamed everything and everybody, but myself most of all, for Gary's illness and death.

I drank a lot, it's true, but I stayed sober enough, when it was necessary, to see that the kids were fed and that they got home safely from school.

Nothing is more ugly than the female alcoholic. And that is what I was turning into, the dreaded stereotype of the *shikker*. Breakfast was vodka and a cup of coffee. Lunch was a bottle of cheap wine. Period. Somehow I got the nerve to drive a car. Somehow I managed to stay alive. Just barely. With the alcohol came a terrible self-hatred. I was ashamed of my drinking.

I was a madwoman after Gary died. I walked around in the rain. I would come home with drenched clothes and wet hair and fall asleep without changing. I collected traffic tickets as one collects souvenirs. It was a miracle that I didn't get arrested for drunk driving.

Friends and relatives kept calling me and sending cards. But their kind words only reminded me of Gary's death. I loathed their sympathy. I wanted no part of them. The only company I craved was my bottle and sometimes a few pills as a chaser.

When the phone rang, I wouldn't answer it. I had my kids tell callers I was unavailable. The only place I went was the grocery store. I'd go to the store in the evenings, get a basket and start pushing it down the aisles, hoping I wouldn't run into anyone I knew, because they'd come up to tell me how sorry they were that Gary died, and I'd start crying again. I'd shop with my head down, not daring to look up for fear I'd see someone I knew. I'd put bananas and milk and cereal in the cart and my legs moved me around, but my mind was elsewhere.

As I'd stand in the checkout line, I'd look around, bewildered, and wonder what the hell I was doing there, buying food, when Gary was dead.

One day I was supposed to attend a parent-teacher conference for Paul at the kids' school, and I felt I had to go. I didn't drink that morning because I didn't want the teacher to think me a lush. As I approached the school, I saw the swings that Gary had played on, and then I caught sight of Gary's second-grade teacher. My heart began to pound, things went black, and I collapsed on the playground. Someone called an ambulance and I found myself in a hospital with a doctor asking questions.

"Did you ever feel like this before? Did you ever have epilepsy?"

I screamed at him, "No, and I never lost a child before either."

It would have been nice if I could have been the brave, strong mother, the heroine, who could say to her family, "Now, it's going to be hard on us, losing Gary, but he's with God in heaven now, and he's a lot better off there. We'll all have to keep a stiff upper lip and go on living. Gary would have wanted it that way."

But that was bullshit. Pure unadulterated bullshit. Gary was dead. That's all there was to it. I could feel no other way than wretched.

Sometimes during that period Jack played the role of a father. He took the kids out to eat and even took them to the movies a few times.

In the background, as he buttoned a jacket for David or answered a question of Paul's, I would hear him whisper, "Ask your mother to go with us."

I would suck in my breath and go for the bottle.

I needed so desperately to talk to someone about Gary and I tried to talk to Jack. He listened a few times, but then he said that talking wouldn't bring Gary back. I knew that, but I still needed to talk.

"Bernice, there's no use talking about Gary. He's dead. It's over and done with."

I made a futile gesture with my hands. "Over and done with?" I screamed. "Are you nuts? It'll never be over and done with."

I wanted to claw at him, to strike him, to shake some feelings into him, but I didn't have the strength. What was the use, anyway?

When I wouldn't speak to people who called, I'd hear Jack say, "I can't understand it. Bernice just isn't Bernice anymore."

Damn it, I'd think. What's the matter with him? How does he expect me to be? How does he expect me to feel?

Am I crazy or is he? One of us is, and I'm not sure which.

A few times he'd talk to me about my drinking, "Bernice, people will think you're an alcoholic. Stop drinking."

"You're the right person to talk, huh?" I said wearily. "The guy who has all the right in the world to tell someone else what they're doing wrong. Don't tell me what to do, Jack. Not ever. Not ever again. And for your information, I don't give a shit what people think anymore."

Didn't he realize that I had to get rid of the solid, sickening ache in my heart or I'd go out of my mind, if I hadn't already?

Friends told me Jack had choked up and cried at Gary's funeral, that he could barely recite the Kaddish, the Jewish requiem for a dead son. In a way I wish I'd been there to see that. Maybe we could have thrown our arms around each other and felt something together for once. But I think that was a rare, overwhelming moment for Jack, and he never displayed such emotion again.

The real seriousness of Jack's disease—the gambling virus—became clear shortly after Gary died. One day when David was going through some papers in a box kept in the bottom drawer of a desk in the den, he came across a bank book. He brought it to me, and I was shocked to find that Jack had his own savings account with $6,500 in it. The money had been deposited both before and after Gary's death.

And he'd let me borrow the money to bury Gary! A lousy $465 was all we needed and Jack asked me to borrow it from his boss. He had felt too awkward himself to ask for the money, so he had me do it. And all the time he had had $6,500 stashed away. Then he had had the gall to take the $465 insurance check!

I was stunned. We had been struggling for dollars to help Gary fight leukemia and Jack had held out all that money for his gambling. At the moment I hated him too much ever to forgive him.

When I confronted him with the bank book, Jack

became angry and refused to discuss it. I was too exhausted and grief-stricken to pursue the matter. Besides, nothing could affect me for long. I just went back to the comfort of my bottle.

I began to have a compulsive need to go to the cemetery. I went every day some weeks, never less than three or four times a week. I used to talk to Gary, pour out the feelings I could not share with Jack. I'd sit in front of Gary's crypt and talk to him in my head. Then I'd drive home, tears streaming down my cheeks, praying aloud that a car would crash into me head-on and put me out of my misery.

Gary's illness left us $11,000 in debt. I knew it would take a lifetime to pay that. At first I spent time trying to make the doctors, nurses, and hospital administrators understand that I could only pay so much every month. But after I'd been yelled at and demeaned often enough, I gave up. "So put me in debtor's prison," I screamed back at them. "I'll pay you what I can afford. If you don't like that, it's too bad."

I found out later that the reason I didn't get too much back-talk on that point was that I was within my legal rights. Paying what you can afford is all that the law demands.

Catastrophic illnesses have broken more homes than earthquakes and floods. The Red Cross and government agencies come around with assistance after natural disasters, but nobody bails you out of your huge, unpayable hospital and doctor bills. Once the government planned a giant crash program to combat cancer, heart disease, and strokes. But the plan was set aside because of our huge expenses in Vietnam.

Someday, I hope the average family will be protected— not just against the medical bills, but against the diseases themselves.

# Chapter 6

AFTER GARY DIED, I stayed in his room a good deal of the time. I left it exactly as it had been the last time he'd been home. His stuffed pink poodle on the bed, his comb and brush on the dresser, on his desk the hand he'd modeled in clay at school, and two report cards—only two, but good ones. There were packages of seeds on his dresser and an assortment of Elvis Presley records.

I used to close the door to his room—it had a little sign taped on it which read "Doctor is out—be back at one o'clock." I'd lie on his bed, searching the blank ceiling for clues. I couldn't pray to a God who would allow such a thing to happen, so I used to hold conversations with Papa.

Why, Papa? Why did Gary die? Was it my fault?

Classic Jewish guilt. Jewish hell. Classic mother guilt. All mothers have it, I think. If our kid dies, we're sure it's our fault. Maybe it is.

What did I do wrong, Papa?

Papa was always telling me, "Something never comes from nothing. Something always comes from something." That was his profound way of saying there's a reason for everything.

Why did my son get leukemia and die? I probed the deepest corners of my mind.

Was it something in our family? I mean, was it hereditary? An individual can be predisposed to illness before birth.

Was it something I did? Was it somewhere we went? Was it just fate? What exactly was it that caused Gary's leukemia?

Am I guilty, Papa? Tell me . . . Please!

When I was pregnant with Gary, I got pernicious anemia. Pernicious anemia stems from a deficiency of vitamin B12. The body may take in enough of the vitamin, but it is unable to absorb and utilize it.

I was given vitamin B12 shots and put on a diet rich in iron to curb the illness. But I didn't follow the doctor's orders. The one time I should have done what he said, I didn't. I was a smartass. Bagels, coffee, and cigarettes were the mainstays of my diet, and when I was in my sixth month, it looked as though I might miscarry. My obstetrician from Beverly Hills prescribed a synthetic hormone known as DES—Diethylstilbestrol.

While Gary was suffering and I was reading like a maniac on leukemia, I discovered that in the 1940s doctors began prescribing DES for pregnant women in the belief that the hormone would reduce the risk of miscarriage. It later came to light that DES definitely has carcinogenic effects on the offspring of those mothers.

My God, had a doctor prescribed a drug that could cause cancer? And had the hormone that I had taken to save me from miscarrying killed that same infant at a later date?

Later I learned that there is evidence that a vitamin B12-folic acid deficiency in the mother may be involved in impairing the immune-disease fighting system of her children. That might explain why some children are more susceptible to disease than others. And scientists have also discovered that there is a relationship between what a mother eats during pregnancy and her children's resistance to infection and disease, even long after they are born. But Papa, I didn't know that then. I would have done things differently, had I known.

Papa, in 1957, when Gary was only three months old, Jack and I went to Vegas, near where the government was doing some nuclear bomb testing. I told Jack that I had read it was unsafe to take the children there, especially an infant. But Jack laughed it off, saying, "Come on Bernice. It's silly to worry. Why do you have to spoil things by worrying? You're supposed to have a good time in Vegas. You read too damn much for your own good."

I was worried about the trip because I had read that nuclear testing could cause cancer or leukemia, particularly in infants, because they are more sensitive to radiation than adults—their immune system is not yet fully operating. What about all those "survivors" of Hiroshima and Nagasaki who developed the disease many years after being exposed to the radioactive blast?

Papa, I knew it was wrong to go there. And yet I went to please Jack. Papa, why did I do that?

Is it possible that Gary and many like him have died because our country wanted to make certain we had a more effective bomb than Russia? It never dawned on me then that I could sue the government for contributing to Gary's death. Now it seems that all of us should sue for the radiation dangers we are being exposed to.

And Papa, there were all those antibiotics Gary took for his colds—massive amounts of medication over the months. When Gary's leukemia was diagnosed the doctors asked me if he'd taken a drug called Chloromycetin, which was known to depress the bone marrow. I tried to find out if any of the antibiotics he'd taken had been Chloromycetin, but no one could give me an answer. Some doctors and scientists have expressed the view that antibiotics and other drugs often used against viral infections in children may play a part in transforming a stubborn infection into leukemia.

And those insecticides, those damned insecticides on Laurie's lawn. Insecticides are known to cause cancer, too. And I let my *mizinik* wade through all that DDT, just· to retrieve some baseballs.

And Papa, there was Gary's lousy diet—all that junk food he ate. Health food advocates claim that preservatives and additives are cancer-causers. Why didn't I listen to them?

Papa, I'm tortured by the thought that I should not have taken Gary off the chemotherapy and switched to the Laetrile and cellular therapy. But I felt I had a good reason. I knew that chemotherapy was not a cure, and I was desperate to find one.

Papa, wherever my mind turns, it seems to find reasons for Gary's death that can be traced back to my negligence or ignorance. I'm so tired of living with my guilt. Where can I find forgiveness? Where can I find out what really happened to Gary? When can I stop mourning?

# Chapter 7

NOTHING THAT HAD HAPPENED previously in my life had prepared me to face the death of my beloved child. It is not normal for parents to bury children. It should be the other way around.

When Gary died, it would have been a comfort to believe that death was not the final end, that at some time in the future, I would be with Gary again. But after watching Papa work religion the way he did, praying in the mornings and evenings and conning all the hours in between, I had no faith to sustain me. And I couldn't say to myself, as some people do, that God wanted Gary to be a little angel. Jewish people don't believe in little angels, so that didn't help. Nothing did. Nothing could. Nothing does.

And one day shortly after Gary died, when I was overcome by feelings of guilt, I called Dr. Eisen and told him I wanted to bring Paul in to see him. Actually, I just needed some words of comfort, which Dr. Eisen was very good at giving. He'd been our family doctor since the boys were babies, from polio and tetanus shots to treating Jack for diabetes and gout. He'd given us more than prescriptions and checkups; he'd given us moral support more times than I could count. He was the kind of doctor movies show as the family physician, concerned and dedicated.

But when Gary was sick, Dr. Eisen advised me always in the direction of traditional chemotherapy. Since there was no hope, there was no point in trying something new, according to him. I, of course, disagreed. If there was no hope, why not try everything and anything?

I had gone against Dr. Eisen's advice on several occasions during Gary's illness, and after Gary died, I began to think maybe I should have listened to the doctor. Maybe he and Dr. Hemp were right. Maybe I had shortened Gary's life by switching treatments.

After Dr. Eisen had examined Paul and found absolutely nothing wrong, he looked at me over his glasses and said, "Bernice, why did you really come here this afternoon?"

My lip was trembling and I was fighting back the tears. He knew it. He could probably smell the liquor on my breath, too. He took me into his office where we could talk in private.

"Now, what is it, Bernice?"

I broke down. "I don't know, doctor. I just keep thinking about Gary," I sobbed.

"Bernice, I understand the pain of your loss. But there is nothing you or I can . . . "

"I don't want to hear that, Dr. Eisen. I want to know something. It's something that's been bothering me more than usual lately. I want to know . . . I want to know if I contributed to Gary's death."

"Contributed? What do you mean?"

"When I went to Tijuana with him and took him off the chemotherapy. Would he have lived if I'd left him on the drugs?"

Dr. Eisen folded his hands in front of him and spoke softly, with patience. "Bernice, I guess I must have told you a thousand times that Gary would have died regardless of what we did to try to help him. Leukemia is fatal. It cannot be cured. And you did all you could. But, you asked my opinion, and I'll tell you as I've told you before. I think you just went overboard. Taking Gary to Tijuana for Laetrile was a futile effort. Those treatments weren't proven methods and had no effect on his disease whatsoever."

I began to go over and over why I had done it. I told Dr. Eisen you don't ever give up on a person until he is dead. I had to try everything. I just couldn't sit there and watch my baby die. If only he'd had a bone marrow transplant.

"Bernice, Bernice." Dr. Eisen insisted. "Bone marrow transplants are still in the talking stage, not the doing stage, for heaven's sake."

What was the matter with him? Didn't he read? I explained to him that doctors were experimenting with that treatment all over the world.

But Dr. Eisen just sat there and listened quietly, offering these wonderful words of encouragement at the end of our conversation, "You have a husband who loves you and three children, Bernice. Just remember that and be grateful."

But I didn't feel grateful. Guilty was the only way I could feel. I exaggerated my part in Gary's illness until I loathed myself. Suicide seemed to be a good answer. I told myself that as soon as I had the energy—maybe the following day or week—I would kill myself. I didn't deserve to live, I told myself bitterly. There was absolutely no good reason why I should live.

In the back of my mind, though, I knew there was a reason. My three other sons. I could hear their comings and goings as I lay in Gary's room. They were still alive, my kids. And they needed me.

Then a new terror overtook me. What if another of my

sons were to come down with the disease? They had all lived in the same place, breathed the same air, the same polluted air. Every cough, every cold, every symptom of illness petrified me.

Because I had read so much on leukemia, I thought all kinds of thoughts and imagined all kinds of things. Could leukemia be contagious at some point—perhaps in the viral stage—and if so, how long would it take to pop up again in one of the others?

I went to the library to check on statistics. Were there any families where more than one child in the family had gotten leukemia? Yes, I read, but it was uncommon.

That scared me to death. So what if it was rare? Gary had gotten it. Why not the others?

I was in a torture chamber of hell.

I wanted to tell someone. I wanted to talk my fears out with someone, preferably a medical man. But I couldn't do that. It was as though I were paralyzed. I felt that if I uttered those words aloud, if they actually came out of my mouth, that would make it really happen. So I carried it all inside me.

Somewhere along the line, Papa's superstitions began to haunt me. I felt that if I got close to my sons again, as close as I had been to Gary, that they would be hexed as he had been. I was afraid that God would take another one to punish me. I didn't know what He was punishing me for, unless it was pride. Perhaps I had acted too happy, perhaps my pride in my four wonderful sons had been flaunted too openly.

"Papa, Papa," I kept repeating to myself like a crazy-woman.'You kept telling me I shouldn't show my happiness so much, or I would get a *Kinehora.*"

So I decided I was going to fool God. I stayed away from my sons. I was going to be indifferent to them, I told myself. Not worry about them so much. Not love them so much. Then, if nothing bad happened for a long, long time, I would come out of my cocoon.

"Please," I prayed, "whoever you are up there, put me in a mental institution. Let me be declared insane. Then I'll know the fears and thoughts I have are ridiculous. Then I'll know I'm really off my rocker and those things can't happen. Please let me die. Let the earth swallow me up. Let me drink myself to death. Just stop me from thinking thoughts like that. Please give me cancer so I can die."

Sometimes prayers are answered.

# Chapter 8

THE LUMP I HAD FOUND in my right breast while Gary was sick continued to grow. In July of 1966, it popped out bright, red, and glassy. I chose to ignore it. I was too absorbed in self-pity and depression to pay attention to my physical condition.

I was still drinking then, going about my chores like a robot. One day I stumbled over the coffee table while I was vacuuming and fell flat on my ass.

David came running to the living room to see what had happened. I picked myself off the floor and staggered to the sofa, sitting there with my hand on my throbbing head.

David stared at me. "Whatsa matter, Mom, you okay?"

I sighed and leaned my head back. "I don't know, son. Yeah. I'm okay. Just leave me alone a minute, would you?"

He didn't. He came up close to me and sat down beside me. When I could finally focus on his face, I saw tears in his eyes. "You're thinking about Gary, aren't you?" he asked.

"Son, I'm always thinking about Gary," I replied.

"You act like you loved him more than you do us," he said. He broke down and put his head in my lap, sobbing.

"David, David, it's not that way at all. I love you all the same, but I thought . . ." I stopped myself. How could I possibly explain to a ten-year-old child all the thoughts that were tormenting me—My fear that another of them would get leukemia and die. It would shock him out of his wits. I couldn't do that.

How had I allowed myself to get that much out of control emotionally? How had I allowed those crazy thoughts to get the better of me? I had not liked watching Papa play games with religion. I had not accepted his superstitions. And yet I had begun to behave as if superstition, fear, and guilt ruled my life.

"Bernice," I said, "it's time to clean up your act. Shape up. Stop drinking. It's not going to bring Gary back. And your other sons need their mother." The next day I woke up sober for the first time in a year.

I made arrangements to go to Tijuana to have my breast examined. I was still intrigued with the idea of Laetrile and had read quite a few articles about how it had helped cancer patients. Since I was by that time afraid the lump might be cancer, I decided at the outset to take a different route from traditional therapy if it turned out to be malignant.

However, the doctor in Tijuana, Dr. Ernesto Contreras, told me he didn't think Laetrile would take care of the lump if it were cancer and he advised that I return to Los Angeles for a biopsy.

"First things first," I said to myself, as I drove home across the border.

First I had to make out a will. I had to see that my sons would be protected in case I died. Whether or not the lump in my breast turned out to be malignant, there was still danger in surgery.

If I died, I knew that sooner or later, Jack would remarry. I did not object to the idea, since I knew I really wouldn't have much say about it—being six feet under.

A Margaret Sullivan I wasn't. She's the actress who portrayed a wife dying of cancer in the old movie, *Shed No Tears for Me*. She didn't want her husband and children to shed any tears over her after she died. I wanted Jack and my sons to cry a hell of a lot for me. I wasn't about to set up Jack with another woman like she did. But I wished I could be sure whoever took my place would take care of my kids. I hoped that if my sons ever did have a stepmother, she would be a loving one. But it would be fine with me if the woman showed Jack the same insensivity, lack of feelings, and inconsideration that he showed me over the years. Apparently I had become a yogi in the great far eastern Indian faith, "Just Retribution."

I sat down at the kitchen table with a pen and writing tablet in front of me and wrote, "I, Bernice Wallin, being of sound mind, hereby bequeath my one-half share of property located at.....................to my three sons, Fred Wallin, Paul Wallin, and David Wallin."

I dated it, signed it, stuck it in an envelope and sealed it. On the front of the envelope, I wrote, "To be opened in the event of my death."

If I died on Friday, I'd be buried on Sunday. The house would go up for sale on Monday and be sold by the following Friday. It would be out of escrow thirty days later and Jack's share would be gambled away shortly afterwards. My sons had to be protected.

I walked into the bedroom and placed the envelope in the dresser drawer where I kept important papers. That way, my family would be sure to find the envelope after my death.

Then I made an appointment with a surgeon.

When I went in for the surgery, I knew I might wake up without a breast. But that idea didn't frighten me. I'd lost a son, and no loss could be greater than that. So take the breast; take my head, for that matter. Who cared? That was my attitude.

I did feel funny walking around lopsided. It was inconvenient. And it hurt like hell. But I welcomed the pain. The masochist in me relished every ounce of physical suffering, hoping that it would outweigh the mental anguish and heartache. It never did.

I derived a perverse pleasure in knowing that something had been taken from my own body. It was a small payment I was making for what I felt was my contribution to Gary's illness. It helped ease the guilt. Not completely, but it helped.

Six months after the mastectomy, a large lump came up in my left breast. A mammograph was taken, and I waited impatiently for the results.

I got them from a phone booth outside a gas station. I had been doing errands for Mama and I was so anxious that I phoned the doctor while Mama waited in the car.

"Bernice, I'm afraid your other breast is going to have to come off," the surgeon told me.

"Please doctor, tell me you're kidding."

"No, Bernice, I'm not kidding," he answered calmly. "I've made arrangements for you to go into Mt. Sinai Hospital tomorrow. Check in there before 3 P.M."

I was stunned. And, finally, terribly frightened. I walked back to the car and told Mama what the doctor had said.

"Bossie, don't worry about nothing," Mama said. "I'll take care of everything at home for you. You just rest your mind. God's going to take care of everything."

I had decided long ago that God had forgotten all about the Wallin family. Maybe He was on vacation and didn't have time to take care of us right now. I was going to have to muddle through this thing alone.

The fact that breast cancer strikes more women than any other type of malignancy does not give comfort to the person involved. To lose a breast can be the most terrifying and traumatic experience in a woman's life. Ninety-nine percent of the women afflicted would attest to that. I was that 1% who was not devastated. But no doubt I would have been, had I not already suffered a far greater tragedy. And so I reacted to the second mastectomy much as I had reacted to the first one. It was painful. Indeed it was. But I wasn't concerned how the loss of my breasts affected my feminity. All I could still think about was Gary.

I knew that if anyone was going to be affected by the surgery, it would be Jack. And if it bothered Jack it wouldn't really matter one way or the other to me.

But as it turned out, it didn't seem to affect Jack either. Or if it did, I never knew about it. And after I healed we had sex as usual. But I was curious. I still wanted to hear how he felt making love to a wife who had no breasts. I tried to talk to him about it. But he wasn't interested in talking. I wanted him to look at the scars or the way the surgery had left me, but he refused to look. I wanted some kind of reaction out of him, some show of emotion, some something. But there was nothing.

And the more he refused to discuss it, the more I questioned and prodded him. Sadistically, perhaps, I was hoping that he would at last be affected by something in our relationship—his pleasures, something that concerned him directly. Who knows? Maybe I wanted in my own way to turn him off sexually as he had turned me off by being insensitive to me and our family's needs.

He'd always been quiet, Jack. And shy. But when I met him, I welcomed his almost humble ways. He was so different from Papa, who seemed loud and obnoxious to me by the time I was a teenager. Papa was always looking for an argument. Jack would do anything to avoid conflict.

Papa happened to think Jack was the greatest. Jack was

the son of one of Papa's business acquaintances and when Papa heard that this son had just returned from the service with $25,000 he'd won gambling, well, Papa didn't hesitate to set us up.

Yet I can truthfully say it wasn't all Papa's doing that made me marry · Jack. There was definitely chemistry there. He was so handsome, I almost had to catch my breath the first time I saw him. He wasn't really tall—about five feet nine inches—but solidly built: big arms, small waist, and coal black hair with a touch of premature gray at the temples. The bluest eyes imaginable. And that nose. Straight and even. I've always been a sucker for a beautiful nose.

Jack had just returned from the army. There was romance in the air and the courting began. Jack did all the little things that young girls go crazy for. He opened doors for me and brought me gardenias. He was gentle and seemed to have the humility my father lacked. And above all, he was honest.

But even then, there was one small thing about Jack that disturbed me—his gambling. It bothered Mama, too. But to her it was no small thing. "Don't marry Jack, Bossie. Gamblers don't make good husbands," she admonished.

But Papa interceded as usual. "Leave her alone, Shifra. Jack is a nice clean-cut Jewish boy. Besides, look at his family. They're good people. His mother Elsie spends her time raising money for the City of Hope and she is a big wheel in the Hadassah. His father owns a pants manufacturing business. What more do you want for your daughter? Be quiet, Shifra. Jack will make a good husband for Bossie. After the children start coming, Jack will stop gambling. Don't worry."

So what if he gambled. He wanted to set up house. Support me. Be my man.

And poof, there went my dreams of becoming a journalist. I'd studied journalism in college and had dreams of riding around on a white horse battling injustice and exposing corruption.

I remember that even as a very small child I marched in protest of Hitler's persecution of the Jews. As a child I probably wasn't even sure why I was marching. Was I really conscious of the ugly philosophies of the Nazis and their inhumane treatment of the Jewish people? Maybe I was just attracted by the glory of crusading. I certainly hope not. But always in my dreams I saw myself as a Dorothy Kilgallen or someone like her.

Yet when Jack came along, my whole perspective changed. I wanted to marry him and have his children.

So that's what we did. We got married, Jack got a job as a butcher, and we started a family.

But I had never asked Jack if he really wanted children. I'd just assumed that every man wanted to be a father as much as I wanted to be a mother. It had never occurred to me that some men are not cut out to be fathers, let alone husbands.

Jack played the new-father role to the hilt. He stood in front of the nursery window and oohed and aahed over each of his newborn sons. He bounded into my hospital room with a big happy grin on his face, carrying a bouquet of flowers. He passed out cigars to his friends, my friends, our friends, to anyone and everyone. But his responsibility ended there.

But sex was good with him. We got along fantastically from the start. For a long time the quality of our lovemaking gave me hope. We achieved physical closeness. Should mental and emotional closeness be so hard to achieve? Unfortunately it was.

Finally I realized that while a climax was nice, it wasn't all there was to marriage. It didn't pay the electric bill or even narrow the yawning abyss between us. Too late I realized you should get to know someone before you marry and jump into bed with him. Too late I realized what it takes to make a marriage.

But should I complain? He never beat me. Although we never had any cash and we were always in debt, there was always plenty of food on the table.

And Jack never fooled around with other women. I should be grateful for that, shouldn't I? I knew the only other women he was interested in were the four ladies who lived within the pack of playing cards.

Perhaps the real problem was that our goals were as far apart as they could have been. I didn't want a mansion. Just a house with a backyard, for God's sake. I didn't want a Cadillac. I just didn't want to have to worry about whether or not my car was going to make it around the block.

And I wanted a little more money for the boys. I wanted them to have nice clothes, a decent place to bring their friends. But Jack didn't care about any of those things. He would have been content living in an orange crate as long as he could gamble.

Jack wanted to keep renting. But by the time Gary came along, I insisted on buying a house. Why make the landlord rich, I argued? Build an equity in our own home. So I went househunting alone. I walked my legs off looking for a house that would fit our limited budget. I wasn't particularly fussy. I just wanted to get into something that would be ours. I knew I'd fix it up bit by bit as our needs arose.

I wanted to buy a house that was close to UCLA. I knew college was a long way off for the boys, but I believed in planning ahead. I finally found a house in Culver City that would do—1,050 square feet in all, but I loved it. The size of the rooms didn't matter. It's true, they were minscule, but it was a start and I was grateful. Jack didn't see the house until the day we moved in.

The thing that hurts me most about Jack is that his great potential went unused. He has a quick mind, a sense of humor, wit and charm. I couldn't understand why he didn't use them to make a better life for himself, for me, and for his children.

Jack gambled and made some big money now and then, but I never saw much of it. It was always poured right back onto the gambling tables. And because I had been so used to the wheeling-dealing of my father, it had never occurred to me that Jack would not also have that kind of ambition and drive. But the only place where I saw ambition was in his gambling, always looking to make that "Big Score."

The distance between us grew over the years until there was a horrible emptiness. The loneliness was unbearable at times.

So maybe I should have left him. But I kept putting it off. I found all kinds of excuses for not leaving. I just kept hoping he would eventually start taking an interest in his family. I kept telling myself I'd wait until the kids were grown. I'd wait until the bills were paid or until I got some more schooling so I could get a good job.

But by the time I'd had my mastectomies, I was trapped. I couldn't leave. But it wasn't the lack of my breasts that stopped me from taking my sons and walking out. I was just physically and emotionally drained from all the heartache and sickness and it seemed far too late and too difficult for me to start a new life somewhere. And the thought of remarrying frightened me. There was always the possibility of another Jack. So I simply took the line of least resistance and stayed.

# Chapter 9

After my second mastectomy, doctors told me that by 1971, if there was no recurrence of cancer in my body, I could consider myself cured.

During that five-year period I continued to cater to my family and grieve for Gary. The boys were all teenagers by then. Fred had grown long hair and a beard, Paul was playing basketball, and David was already into his Elvis Presley imitations.

I suppose, to some degree, I was concerned about the possibility of cancer returning. Whenever I felt a pain somewhere in my body, my heart must have skipped a beat or two, but I never really worried about myself and I tried not to worry the rest of the family.

I had seen Gary die right in front of my eyes and gone through cancer surgery and yet I couldn't imagine myself dying. Deep down I was probably frightened, but the fear never came into my consciousness. It didn't prey on my mind—but it must have been there. Besides, even if I wasn't a believer, I couldn't believe that the man upstairs would inflict me with any more tsuris. Stupid?

I never held back from my kids the fact that I had cancer and that my breasts had been removed. You can't hide something like that from your family. "The way I see it," I told the boys when they asked me, "I'm like a person who lost her arms or legs in a train wreck or a car accident." They accepted that explanation.

I can't count the times I've walked out of the house without my falsies, looking like a young boy on top. I never wore a padded or inflated bra anywhere unless I felt like it and I didn't put one on so I could disguise the fact that I had no breasts. When I went anywhere special, I put my falsies on, but only if I wanted to and could find them. I was constantly misplacing or losing them.

At first I tried to tell myself I was going to the library or the market minus the falsies because I didn't give a damn about myself or how I looked. Then I tried to make myself believe that it was because the cheap brassieres I could afford were uncomfortable. And then I came to the revelation that I must have some Bella Abzug and Gloria Steinem in my makeup. Pre ERA, but still twenty years too late, I decided that I was going to be my own person.

I realized I was angry—frightfully angry and defiant. I was belligerent and ready to fight at the slightest provocation. Not that I looked for a fight but I was ready to fight back if anyone started something. Before I had trembled at the harsh words of a bill collector; now the same person cringed at my caustic words. This was an entirely new ball game for me; I wanted to strike out at anyone who infringed upon my rights.

For example, there was the time Jack bought me a huge oak planter for Mother's Day from Two Guys Department Store. It was pretty but I decided to exchange it for whatever I found there that I liked better.

The store manager informed me politely that plants were not exchangeable.

"Since when?" I asked courteously.

"We do not exchange plants." he said, ignoring my question.

"Since when?" I repeated.

"I don't know since when. But this is our policy," he said.

"Sir, I must have an exchange. I do not need this plant and I'd like to buy something else, preferably a pants suit for myself."

"I'm sorry, but that's impossible."

For a moment, I thought of myself as Gregory Peck in *Gentlemen's Agreement,* trying to get a room in a restricted hotel. I wasn't going to take anything from anyone.

"Why is it impossible?" I asked quietly. I looked carefully around the store, my eyes focusing on the two windows facing the street.

"We have our store policy that we abide by."

"Sir," I said slowly as I pointed to the windows, "which window would you prefer that I throw this plant out of?"

You're not supposed to end a sentence with a preposition, Bernice, I thought to myself as I watched the calm expression on the man's face turn to one of utter amazement. He stared at me intently as he said, "Wait here a moment, please. I'll come back with a refund slip."

He was back in a matter of seconds, but not with a refund slip. I knew he had bypassed all the store regulations when he handed me the $21 and some change. "Here you are," he said. "Buy whatever you wish."

I took the money and watched him walk away shaking his head and probably thinking, "What a crazy lady. She's nuttier than a fruitcake. I hope she gets the hell out of here in a hurry."

As I walked away I wondered how many people had accepted his company's rules without questioning them.

I chuckled inwardly—maybe I should have been the poker player in the family—my, oh my, how I had run a good bluff! Or was it?

Right or wrong, nobody was going to screw me around anymore.

"I'll be dammed if I'll wear a padded bra. People will either take me as I am or the hell with 'em," I muttered to myself as I walked home. "I'll go around looking flat-chested as a board if I want to."

In spades, I was telling the world that it had taken my son and my breasts and I was never going to kowtow to it.

Charles Dickens' Tiny Tim repeats over and over, "God bless us every one." My philosophy had become, "Go screw yourself, one and all."

Because David was the youngest and home more than the others, there were many times after my breast surgeries that I was forced to ask him to hook my brassiere, assist me from the bathtub, button the back of a blouse, or perform any number of other functions I was incapable of doing during the crucial times of my illness. He had to see the effects of my mastectomies.

Sometimes I even joked about the loss of my breasts. When I said, "Call me heap strong Amazon lady. Me shoot arrow real straight," the boys knew what I meant. I had shown them a book that said that Amazon women had their right breast ripped off so they could shoot arrows more proficiently. We laughed our heads off one day when Paul brought home a bow and arrow set and put it alongside my dinner plate.

Although I laughed a little now and then, nothing took my mind off Gary's death or my guilt for long. I stopped nagging Jack about his gambling. There was no more arguing, no more talk about improving our home. None of that seemed to matter anymore.

What did begin to matter was stopping the Vietnam

war. Deep inside my heart, I felt that the radiation from bomb testing could have been the major culprit in Gary's death. I was determined that none of my other boys would die fighting needlessly in some foreign country. I resolved not to allow my sons or anyone else's sons to be used as gun fodder in an immoral war to fatten the pocketbooks of profiteers. So I did what I could to help.

Because Senator Eugene McCarthy from Minnesota came out so strongly against the war, I walked blocks getting signatures for him so that he could get his name on the presidential ballot.

I marched in Woman's Strike for Peace demonstrations. I folded letters, sealed envelopes, attended counsel sessions, and sometimes counseled young men who did not want to sacrifice their lives for nothing.

I breathed a deep, deep sigh of relief when the war finally ended.

What I remember most clearly about those five years preceding 1971 is that they were long, lonely, and depressing. Since there was no one to turn to in my despair, I called on my memories of Papa. Although he was physically removed from the world, I knew his spirit was with me.

I didn't know how to apply Papa's philosophy to my own life. By then I thought my life was such a mess it couldn't be remedied. But Papa's way of thinking confirmed what experience had taught me so far: that life is a rough road to travel and you have to watch out for yourself.

By 1971, though, I began feeling better. I knew it was the fifth year the doctors had talked about, and so far no more cancer had been found in my body. I began to feel I'd beaten the damned disease. I felt curiously victorious. Cancer had taken my son and I still felt guilty about that. But gradually reason began to overtake my self-pity. I could see that my other sons really did need me, and I'd given cancer a run for its money this time.

I began to laugh a little more. And for the first time since Gary died, I could mention his name without breaking down. I painted our entire house that year, a room at a time. And I started cooking big meals again. I started listening to music again while I cooked and cleaned.

I even found the initiative to go to a plastic surgeon and have my nose fixed. It's not the greatest nose job in the world, but it made me feel better that I was starting to take pride in my appearance again.

I'll never forget the examination Dr. Eisen gave me at the five-year mark. "You're cured, Bernice," he told me. "You have nothing to worry about."

I bought a bottle of champagne and took it home to my family so we could celebrate.

But cancer has a way of being so viciously secretive. It quietly gnaws. It stealthily devours your insides and sucks your lifeblood dry while you sip champagne and dance a little jig. Soon after that little celebration dinner, I started bleeding profusely because of a number of cysts in my uterus. My periods lasted twenty-four days out of the month and were accompanied by severe cramps. There was no mention of cancer, but Dr. Eisen suggested surgery. I wasn't too crazy about the idea of a hysterectomy and decided to wait to see if it wouldn't stop.

Then in 1972, I detected a pain in my leg, a slight pain at first, just enough to annoy me. I assumed that it was rheumatism or arthritis or something like that and I joked with myself, "Gettin' old, Bernice."

It became a standing joke with all of my friends that I had hurt myself playing basketball. With a houseful of men, sports was at the top of the list, particularly basketball. When one of my friends asked me why I was limping so badly, I responded glibly, "I was going up for a rebound."

When the pain increased, though, and I started limping

around the house all the time, I called Dr. Eisen again. After a perfunctory examination, he prescribed pain killers, confirming my little joke that it must be old age setting in.

For a while the pain went away. But when it came back, even with the pain killers, it was worse. I took more pills. They didn't work. As a matter of fact, the pain began to set other places in my body on fire, until every part of me was hot and sore. I became alarmed.

Finally, Dr. Eisen told me to go into the hospital for tests.

"What could it be?" I asked him nervously.

"Probably not a thing, Bernice, but you'd better have it checked out so we can get rid of that pain for you."

"Come on, doctor. What could it be? You think it's cancer again?"

"Well now, it could be anything, Bernice, but in your case, I hardly think so. It's been five years. I told you."

"I know. I know. I'm cured."

But I didn't want to go into the hospital. I was afraid of what they might tell me. And I was afraid that if I went, I wouldn't be able to dance and sing Mazel Tov at my son Paul's wedding, which was going to take place on July 29.

Fred flew in from his newspaper job in Boston to be best man at Paul's wedding. When we picked him up at the airport, he noticed my limp right away.

"What's the matter, Mom, getting old or something?" he joked.

"That's right, son, over the hill," I said, forcing a laugh. I could tell by Fred's face he was concerned.

He didn't really say anything more to me about it until later that night. I was limping around the kitchen after dinner, washing the dishes, and he leaned against the cabinet, drying each dish slowly and carefully. He watched me intently as we talked. Finally he said, "Mom, what is that limp anyway?"

I tried to seem carefree and unconcerned. I shrugged. "I don't know, Fred. I painted the bathroom last month. Maybe I . . ."

"Last month? What's last month got to do with it?"

"I think I pulled something, that's what."

"And you're still sore? A month later?"

"It hasn't been quite a month," I told him.

"Did you go see Dr. Eisen?"

"I did."

"What did he say?"

"He said it's probably nothing."

"Is that all he said?"

"That's all."

"He didn't want you to get it checked out?"

"Later," I said.

He looked at me dubiously. "Later?"

"Yes. Later. After the wedding."

"Promise?"

I wanted to break down and cry on his shoulder. But I just said, "I'm going already. What do you want me to do? Sign it in blood?"

Paul's wedding took place on July 29, 1972, a hot summer night. I walked into the synagogue wearing a filmy blue thing some salesgirl had picked out for me. I hadn't felt like shopping and had simply asked a cute blond salesgirl at the Broadway Department Store what she thought would be good for a wedding—my son's—and when she pulled out the blue dress, I just said, "I'll take it."

I left the big shoulder strap bag filled with Tampax and Kotex in the coat room of the synagogue with my coat and a change of underwear. By that time, the bleeding was so bad that I had to change every half hour or less.

I didn't look exactly ravishing at my son's wedding. I was quickly degenerating. I looked twenty years older than my age and I hobbled like a hag.

I had to sit with my dress kind of pulled up around my

waist so that I wouldn't bleed all over myself. I was afraid to stand up for fear my dress would be stained. Every few minutes I had to run to the rest room to check.

The pain in my body was intense. I throbbed every-where. It was worse that night than it had ever been.

But despite the agony inside my body, my heart trembled with joy as Paul walked down the aisle with his bride, Sharon. Paul—my second son, but the first to marry. Barely twenty and taking a wife. It was one of the proudest moments of my life. Paul was attending UCLA and would soon go to law school. I knew he would do well.

Mama was there that night. If only Papa could have seen how beautiful she looked as she walked down the aisle, he would have been so proud. She stood straight and erect in her royal blue gown and silvery white crown of thick, wavy hair. She looked so regal, so splendid. I looked twice her age, my body bent, my face wrinkled, sunken, and drawn.

When it was time for Jack and me to walk down the aisle, Jack had to hold my arm tightly so that I wouldn't fall. I had found that by turning my foot over to one side when I walked, it relieved the pain somewhat. But I looked like a cripple waddling down the aisle, trying to hold up my head and smile.

The wedding was beautiful. Sharon's parents are Se-phardic Jews, so the ceremony was held in the garden of a beautiful Sephardic synagogue.

As we stood under the *chupa,* the traditional Jewish canopy, the rabbi, following the Sephardic custom, wound the long, fringed prayer shawl—the *tallis*—around Paul and Sharon. Then they sipped in turn from a wine glass and the rabbi said, "Just as it takes a long time for the wine to find its flavor, so it takes two people a long time to develop the full savor of their relationship."

The wine glass was then wrapped in a towel and placed on the ground, where Paul stepped on it. The rabbi continued, "May the number of pieces into which this shatters symbolize the many years that you will spend together."

And then came the music! Such glorious music! Chassen, Kalleh, Mazel Tov—Chassen, Kalleh, Mazel Tov.

Watching Sharon and Paul recite their marriage vows, so young and full of innocent anticipation, I thought of my own wedding twenty-five years ago and how I had looked forward to such happy years.

I glanced at Jack several times during the ceremony. The years had been kind to him. He was still a good-looking man for his fifty-four years. True, he had gained a paunch over the years, and his gray hair was thinning out, but he still had that ruddy complexion, his handsome nose and the cleft chin. Ah yes, the cleft chin. Each of our sons had Jack's cleft chin, the Wallin trademark.

I felt a thrill of pride as I gazed at each of my six-foot sons who stood engrossed in the solemnity of the occasion. How they had grown. Fred, with his deep, penetrating eyes; Paul, usually exuberant, now looking so serious; and David, my long-haired one, a flirt with the girls, now trying to be so manly, so earnest.

After the ceremony came the reception. The liquor flowed like water and the food came out on torch-lit trays.

I wanted so much to dance that night. But when Paul asked me, I had to turn him down. The pain was just too much, and I'd been afraid to take any more pain killers, knowing they didn't mix with champagne. I wanted to do the Kisatchki, the Russian dance often done at Jewish and Russian weddings. You get down close to the ground, hop on one foot, and throw the other one out in front. And then there's the Hora, where everyone dances and sings in a circle.

Why was I, the lady with ten or twelve dancing cups at home, sitting there while everyone danced around me? It seemed impossible.

Oh well, I comforted myself, I'll go to the hospital

tomorrow for those checkups on my leg. They'll take care of it for me, and I'll dance at the next wedding of one of my sons. I was pretending I wasn't worried.

Paul and Sharon were off at midnight to honeymoon in San Francisco. By that time I was exhausted and glad to go home. I couldn't help saying as Jack and I drove home that I hoped Paul would drive carefully and that everything would be okay with them.

Jack laughed. "He's got another woman to take care of him now, Bernice. You can stop worrying."

Never.

I sighed and leaned my head against the cold vinyl head rest. Fred would be returning to his job in Boston. David would soon be going away to college. I would miss the comings and goings of my sons and their friends. The house would be so quiet.

# Chapter 10

I CHECKED INTO the Cedars of Lebanon Hospital in Hollywood the day after Paul's wedding. The pain in my leg by this time was unbearable.

How I hated hospitals. I'd had my fill of them. And yet there I was again. I seemed doomed to a life chained to some hospital bed.

The tests began on Monday. Hours and hours of tests. Three complete days of tests. Blood tests, bone scans, brain scans, liver scans, and x-rays.

"Please try not to move. Lie very still. Hold your breath. Now let it out. Thank you. Now we'll just do a couple more." The voices of those testers were always so crisp and cool, the voice you'd expect a robot to have.

For the bone scans, radioactive material was injected into a vein of my arm, and then about an hour later, the scanner moved slowly across my body, recording the findings on film. Then the pathologist studied the scan to see if there was a concentration of the material in a particular area.

When the technicians started repeating the x-rays and scans, I sensed that something was radically wrong.

Sitting there humbly in my white hospital gown, I studied their facial responses to my tests. "Can't you tell me what you see?" I asked them meekly.

"You know only your doctor can give you the results, Mrs. Wallin." They were polite but firm.

Well, it wasn't hard for me to figure out. What else could it be? After all, when you have excruciating pain, it means something is pretty wrong with you. And I was scared. I knew that cancer spreads like wildfire if there is even one malignant cell left after surgery. Maybe they hadn't gotten it all out of my breasts. Maybe it was all over my body by now.

I was positive that the pain in my leg was a symptom of a metastasis. That's the word used to refer to malignant cells, breaking off from the primary site and migrating to other parts of the body. A metastasis. I was expecting to hear that word from one of the doctors any minute.

There were lots of visitors during those first three days, both friends and family. David and Fred came with cheery news about what was happening at home, in the neighborhood, how the fish in our aquarium were doing, how my plants were doing, what Mama was up to, gossip, anything. I bantered with them, pretending I wasn't terrified.

To be honest, I didn't like people flocking to my bedside. I didn't let on or anything, but I wished they'd all go away. I kept thinking, they're lying to me, every one of them. They all know something I don't. I'll bet anything I'm terminal and everyone's merely humoring me. Look at the way they watch me—all that compassion and sympathy. As if to say, "Poor Jack, what's he going to do after she's gone?"

I watched them all so carefully when they came to see

me, trying to get behind their smiles and words to see what they were trying to hide from me. I tried to trip them up in conversation so they'd spill what they knew. Then, in a fit of complete paranoia, I began picturing them standing around my coffin. "That's how they'll look," I thought to myself, watching them group around my bed.

My reaction to the disease this time was a little different from my reaction to the breast cancer, when Gary's death was still fresh in mind. Now I had more desire to live. I still mourned for my son, I still had pangs of guilt; but I had by this time convinced myself that life was precious, and that I had not done enough with mine. So many things to do, so many things left undone. I was holding onto my life with a firmer grip. I wasn't ready to let it slip away. Not yet.

The question "Why me?" was now constantly on my mind. I went through severe attacks of self-pity and found myself crying in the middle of the night, from both physical pain and resentment. The only way I could stop those crying spells was to get angry with myself. Oh what a martyr you are, Bernice, I reprimanded myself sternly. You'd better stop or you'll drive yourself crazy. Quit sobbing in your beer, I told myself. You'll find out what's what soon enough.

On the third night, in the middle of my hospital dinner, after all the scans and x-rays had been taken and read by the pathologist, Dr. Eisen strolled leisurely into my room, looking just as he always did—calm, cool, and relaxed.

I was buttering a slice of rye bread, but I dropped it when I saw him amble in, his hands stuffed deep into the pockets of his blue jeans. He was wearing a yellow T-shirt, and I thought it looked ridiculous for a bald-headed man Dr. Eisen's age to be wearing a yellow T-shirt. Especially a doctor in a hospital. But in a way, it was comforting to see him looking so casual. It took some of the urgency out of the situation.

"How are you feeling, Bernice?" he asked, coming close to my bed and patting my hand.

"How should I feel?"

"That's right, answer a question with a question." He smiled pleasantly.

"You want to know how I feel? I feel like a pin cushion with all the shots I get around here, if you want to know. God, they make me groggy. A nurse comes in, stabs me in the butt, and then I'm out like a light. It's ridiculous." I was making small talk, chattering inanely. I knew there was something unavoidable we must discuss, but I wanted to put it off. I picked up my rye bread and took a bite. It was like trying to swallow a piece of cardboard. I gulped some water. It didn't help.

Dr. Eisen hadn't always been bald-headed, but he'd always had those compassionate blue eyes. That night they weren't sparkling as they usually did. He peered at me over his glasses. "You look fine," he said.

"Yeah, I look gorgeous," I retorted. "So tell me. What's the story? What did the tests show, Dr. Eisen?"

He took a deep breath. "Well, from your x-rays and scans, we do see a higher uptake in the left iliac region, Bernice. There's a large spot on your hipbone."

I coughed nervously and toyed with my wedding band. "Yeah? Go on."

"The ilium is the haunch bone that forms a joint with the sacrum, but well, I guess you know that with all the reading you've done."

I nodded.

"There's a six-millimeter nodule overlying the fourth anterior rib. Nothing can be done about that at present. Dr. Cohan, the orthopedic specialist, will do a bone biopsy on the suspected area, and if the sample proves malignant, Dr. Meadows, your surgeon, will perform a total hysterectomy."

I winced.

"Well, Bernice, you know removal of the female organs cuts down the estrogen supply, and we think estrogen is very instrumental in the spread of cancer. And removing the estrogen has been helpful in controlling cancer for a short period. You know that?"

"So you think it's cancer," my voice trembled. "It's a metastasis, isn't it, Dr. Eisen?"

"We have to check it out, Bernice," he said. "But after looking at the x-rays and some of the scans, I have to say there is a good chance that cancer is there. I've always been honest with you, and I'm not going to stop now. I want you to be aware of what's happening to you." He tilted his head slightly and winked at me. "I'm sure with all you've read on cancer, you know pretty much what's happening anyway. But I don't want you torturing yourself. I've scheduled surgery for tomorrow morning. Nursing has been informed not to give you any more to eat or drink this evening. The anesthetist will be in to see you shortly. Any questions?"

I shook my head. So soon. So soon, this surgery? Why so soon?

"We want to determine what your pain is all about," he answered my silent question. "And speaking of pain, Bernice, I see from your chart that you're asking for pain killers more often than the four-hour period I prescribed. Is the pain getting worse?"

"Pretty bad, doctor. Kind of hard to take."

"Well, you know when you get the hysterectomy, the pain may be relieved for a while," he reminded me. "Maybe this operation will help you. I surely hope so. Now, listen, I'll see you after the surgery. Good luck."

As he turned to leave, he added, "I forgot to ask about Paul's wedding."

"It was a lovely wedding." I forced the hint of a smile. The pain was excruciating.

The door closed behind him. And there was silence.

Solid, frightening silence, except for the droning sound of a night moth fluttering against the screen trying to get in.

I felt drained. I knew I wouldn't be able to handle visitors, not even my own family, so I picked up the phone and called home.

David answered, out of breath. "What's up, Mom? How are you feeling?"

"I'm all right, son, but Dr. Eisen just told me I get operated on tomorrow morning, and I'm pretty tired this evening, so maybe it'd be better if I didn't have any company tonight. Now put your grandmother on the phone for a minute before I talk to your father."

"Bossie? Bossie? What is it?" Mama's voice crackled over the wire.

"Mama, please don't buy chocolate cookies or any kind of chocolate candy," I told her. "David's allergic to chocolate."

"I know that, Bossie, why are you telling me?"

"And listen, Mama, don't wear yourself out. They're not children any more. They're grown men. Ask Sally to drive you to your doctor so you can keep your appointment. It looks like I'll be in the hospital for the next week or two."

"Well, what is it? How are you feeling?"

I sighed. Everyone was always asking me how I was feeling. I felt lousy. "Fine, Mama, don't worry about anything. Now let me talk to Jack."

"We were just starting for the hospital when the phone rang. Are you okay?" Jack asked.

"Yes, everything's okay," I lied. "But I'm really tired, Jack, and my surgery is scheduled for tomorrow morning. I'd just rather you didn't come over tonight."

"What? Why not?"

"I'm just tired, that's all, Jack. I'll see you after the surgery."

"What time is the surgery?"

"Early. I don't know." I was becoming annoyed. I wanted off the phone. I wanted to be alone.

"Bernice. You sure you don't want me to come over tonight?"

I could almost hear him making plans in his head to shoot out to Gardena. His mecca. A big lump formed in my throat. I was either going to break down and cry or throw up. "Look Jack, from the way Dr. Eisen was talking tonight, it must be cancer. Now I'd . . . like to hang up. Good-by, Jack."

I hung up, leaned back against the pillows and glanced around the room. It was small and square and stifling. Everything was chrome and white and clean. Blindingly clean.

So tomorrow surgery, I told myself. Tomorrow I find out whether I live or whether I die.

# Chapter 11

THE MORNING OF MY SURGERY, I woke up with that blasted pain all over again and my heart racing a mile a minute.

A blinding whiteness washed the entire sky with that nondescript haze so well known in Southern California. The venetian blinds formed the sunlight into thin, transparent slabs, while dust specks, thick and heavy, wandered from one stream of light to the next.

My mind was blank. Damn, I couldn't think. I was trying hard to think. I wondered what time it was. I wondered if the Dodgers had won last night. I wondered what my family would fix for dinner that night.

The night before, when I had spoken with Dr. Eisen, all I could think of was the cancer. Was it cancer? Was it going to be terminal? Would I turn into a vegetable? Would I die a painful death? All these thoughts overshadowed the real surgery I might be facing—the removal of the female organs.

The morning light was barely showing itself and already I was depressed. I reached over to the bedside table and switched on my transistor radio. I wanted to listen to the news. Maybe the horrors of the world around me would take my mind off my own troubles.

The nurse came in, all cute and cheery. Sometimes I hated that kind of nurse. Was I jealous? Yes, but not of her nice figure or her pretty face. It was her vitality I envied, her good health.

As she came in she asked me that now tiresome question, "How are you feeling?" I think I snapped something sarcastic at her and later apologized. That was a pretty familiar behavior pattern of mine for a while.

After she'd taken my pulse and temperature and scribbled a few things on her chart, she handed me a pile of surgical garb and told me to put them on.

I always looked so wretched before surgery. Those absurd green hospital gowns, that ruffled cap you have to wear, with booties to match. Someone should hire a good clothing designer for these hospitals. No one should have to go to surgery looking like Raggedy Ann.

Staring at my face in the mirror, I wondered who that ugly thing staring back at me was. The person with the dark circles, the lines, the sunken cheeks, the dull, reddish eyes. Whose face could that be? Certainly not mine. I had once won third place in a Queen Esther Beauty Contest at a synagogue in Hollywood. I was a pretty red-haired thing, full of life and joy, a line of beaux forming behind me.

I went back to bed and slumped there like a limp rag doll, watching through my tears the rays of sun that slipped past the curtain and fell across the floor. I felt small, shrunken, and shriveled.

"Time for your drying-up shot, Mrs. Wallin." There was that nurse again, talking like she was about to give me a chocolate sundae instead of one of those miserable shots that dry up the body fluids to keep you from gagging or vomiting during surgery. I didn't need any drying-up shot. I already felt dried up.

Then she gave me a relaxant, put her things back on the cart and wheeled it out, passing Jack as he came shuffling through the door. I watched my husband enter with a dozen roses in his hands. I looked at his face, the familiar smile, and thought, "Bernice, he's great on the social amenities. He always knows when to bring flowers, but that's all he knows. You're in this alone, and don't you forget it."

Jack sat down on the edge of my bed and started making small talk.

"How are you feeling, Bernice?" Original question.

"Fine," I sighed.

"Good. Good." He stared at me blankly.

I stared back at him. I was not going to make it easy for him. I was not going to do the chattering that would take our minds off the real business at hand. I was always the initiator of the conversations. I let him sweat a minute or two.

He finally found his tongue and began to ramble aimlessly about work and home and Mama and some ball game.

I wanted to tell him how scared I was that they'd find cancer, how scared I was of dying. But I knew it was pointless. I knew he didn't want to hear it. I wanted to tell him to be good to our sons. I wanted to talk about Gary, to remind him that Gary had been such a beautiful child. But talking to Jack was a futile exercise. He always acted as if I were speaking some foreign language he didn't understand.

When my head began to whir, I knew the pill was taking effect. I stopped listening to Jack and concentrated on a spot on the ceiling. It looked like a coffee stain and how could there be a coffee stain on the ceiling? I giggled.

"What's so funny?" Jack wanted to know.

"You're just so, so witty," I spluttered. I was really gone.

Two men lifted me onto a gurney, securing my feet and putting a blanket on me. I waved to Jack as I was wheeled down the corridor. He stood in the hallway, waving back like a little boy.

. "Please turn off my transistor, Jack," I said, and felt as if I'd said it in slow motion, as if my speed was 33⅓ rpm instead of my usual 78 rpm.

The pill made my head light. Sensational feeling. I'd make a great junkie . . . loved that feeling . . . when you're going away from yourself, floating somewhere away from your body . . . sleepy, warm . . . comfortable.

I passed through the huge doors of the operating room. My surgeon was waiting for me, dressed in his own hospital ensemble, gloved and masked. "Let's get to work, Bernice," he said.

There was the anesthetist in the background - that nice young man who had come to my room the evening before to ask me if I was allergic to any medication. I tried to say hello to him, to be friendly, but I came off like a sloppy drunk.

He smiled reassuringly and said, "Things will be fine, Bernice."

The enormous overhead lamp seemed huge and grotesque, like something out of a science fiction movie. I was switched from the gurney to the operating table and lay there squinting sleepily up at the harsh, glaring light that looked powerful enough to shine its beam right through me.

The anesthetist searched for a vein. I felt the light prick of a needle. The shapes became blurred. I slipped into unconsciousness. Nestling into oblivion is a good feeling. Then there is no more agony. . . .

As I went further and further under, I wondered, "Can

this be a little like dying? Dying must be like this. When you go to sleep you lie down and close your eyes and after a while you wake up and realize you've been asleep. But when you die you close your eyes and after a while you don't realize anything. Papa died. And he must have felt strange, passing from this side of the world to one with which he was completely unfamiliar. Gary died. I wonder how he felt when he crossed the line. What was he thinking? Where was he, anyway?

After the operation, I was in intensive care for two days, and completely out of it practically the whole time. Oh, every once in a while I'd hear voices. One nurse's voice kept buzzing in my ear, "Cough now, Bernice, cough. Your lungs are filling with fluid, honey, and I want you to cough. If you don't cough, you'll get pneumonia, Bernice. Now, cough."

And then I heard my sister Sally's voice gasping between sobs, "Bossie, cough, dummy! Don't ruin our lives by dying! Cough!

I don't know if I ever did cough for them. I guess I must have. I came out of it and I didn't get pneumonia.

Dr. Eisen says while I was coming out of it, I kept calling out for Papa. He says I kept talking about dancing, about how I wanted to go dancing.

I do remember Dr. Eisen trying to humor me about the dancing. Telling me I'd have to wait a while for that. I tried to explain to him how I'd always loved dancing, how I'd wanted to dance at Paul's wedding, but couldn't. I guess I made no sense at all to the doctor, who kept smiling down at me as if he were humoring a babbling idiot.

I tried to move but couldn't. My left arm was strapped to a board and a needle was inserted into my vein. An IV tube connected to a bottle hanging on a portable chrome stand dripped glucose and water monotonously. I tried to focus on the drops but the concentration nauseated me.

I couldn't talk; my mouth felt parched. I was grateful when a nurse came and swabbed my mouth with a damp gauze on a stick. She gave me a few sips of water, and it tasted better to me than chilled wine from a crystal goblet. I groaned my thanks.

I ached all over. Starched white caps darted everywhere like lines and lines of so many doves flitting through my room.

But finally, on the third day, I began to come out of it. The faint, muted sounds that had sounded garbled and distant for so many days became louder that day.

Someone touched my hand. It was Dr. Eisen taking my pulse.

"Doctor," I whispered weakly, gripping the sheets, my body tensed. "What was it? Was it cancer?" They were the first words out of my mouth, forced out with pain and fear. How frightened I was, how obsessed with my disease.

He didn't answer right away. He made some notes on his chart, puttered around my bed, said something to a nurse.

"Doctor," my voice tried to convey more urgency. Then I realized he was probably stalling, choosing his words. "What was it? What did they find? Tell me."

"Well, of course I'm going to tell you, Bernice," he said, coming up close to me and putting his hand gently on my forehead. "It's a metastasis. Metastasized breast cancer. The bone biopsy confirmed the x-rays. All that pain—it's been caused by cancer. Evidently some of the cancer cells from your breast malignancy entered the bloodstream. Or it could have spread through the lymph glands to the bone."

Did he say cancer? Again? Metastasis? "Are you saying ...do you...do I....do I have cancer again? I can't believe it." Despite the fact that I thought I was ready to hear those words, I felt they couldn't be true. My heart chilled. I had read enough to know that when breast cancer spreads to distant organs, it means death. It's incurable by any present treatments. My hands released their grip on the sheets. I felt my body give way.

I was going to die! I mean *really* die. And not in the remote future. It could be soon. This hit home so hard, I just lay back in my bed and didn't even hear the rest of what Dr. Eisen was telling me. Something about how they would be able to try such and such a treatment on me as soon as such and such a thing was over and things were going to be okay.

Okay? How could he say such an asinine thing? Things hadn't been okay in my life for years. Now I had to face death . . . again.

"Papa, Papa," I cried silently. "I don't want to die. Not yet. I love my sons. I want to see them fulfill their dreams. Please, Papa, if you've still got that pipeline to the man upstairs, tell him to get off my back. I know in every house some rain must fall. But why in the hell does it have to pour in mine?"

Where do you start facing something like that rationally? At first I was panic-stricken, but I kept telling myself to calm down and face it with reason and logic. After all, I wasn't terminal yet. Not yet.

Whoa, Bernice. Cool it. Figure this out.

I could classify myself as having advanced cancer, not terminal. But I knew that once cancer hit one of my vital organs, I'd be considered terminal.

I knew that if it hit my stomach, I wouldn't be able to eat. If it hit my bowels, I wouldn't be able to eliminate. If it infested my lungs and diaphragm, I wouldn't be able to breathe. But worst of all, if it hit my brain, I would be incapable of thinking. To sit, a helpless observer, as the disease made its inroads upon my body would be bad enough. To watch it make its inroads upon my brain would be beyond my endurance.

I cringed at the thought of becoming dependent on others as the disease progressed. I'd need help from Jack or from my sons for the simplest things, like washing my face, fixing a meal, or going to the bathroom. Since my mastectomies, I'd become used to taking care of myself and my family again. And it had always made me uncomfortable to be waited on.

David had been only eleven or twelve at the time of my breast surgeries when I had had to rely on him for help. Now he was a young man, and with Fred and Paul away from home, the whole responsibility would fall upon him. I didn't want him to be burdened with taking care of me again.

As for Jack, how could I count on him to help me? He had never called any of my doctors to check on my physical condition. He would accept my death as impassively as he had accepted Gary's. I remembered that a few days after each of my mastectomies, when I was able to sit up a little, Jack brought to the hospital a brown paper bag filled with unpaid bills and a checkbook. He considered it my job to write the checks—in the hospital or out. Jack simply didn't want to be bothered with anything unpleasant. He had insulated himself from his family and from life. I expected no support from him.

As I lay there trying to come to terms with the reality of my condition, I decided I wasn't ready to die. I hadn't accomplished enough. Even as a child I wanted to make the world remember me. Does every child feel that way? I've often wondered if those are just the fantasies of a potential ego-maniac. But ego-maniac or not, I felt I hadn't yet done the things I was capable of doing.

Before I was married, I dreamed of becoming an investigative journalist. When I married, I changed my mind and decided to be content with having sons. I thought that would fulfill my need for accomplishment. But as much as I had enjoyed motherhood, I felt there was something missing.

I began to outline my battle. Maybe it was a slightly subconscious campaign at the time, but strategies began to formulate.

I knew that there were three established methods of treating metastasized cancer: surgery, radiation, and chemotherapy. I'd already undergone surgery. The breasts were gone, the female organs were gone. What else could they cut off or out?

As for radiation, the object of that is to deliver a lethal dose to the malignancy with a minimum dose to the surrounding tissue and organs. Although cancerous tissue is more susceptible than normal tissue, normal tissue is also affected. So lethal dosage for a malignancy must be balanced against normal tissue tolerance. And in large doses, radiation affects the body as a whole.

The same is true of chemotherapy. Intended to kill cancerous cells, it kills not only the bad, but also good cells, particularly those in the bone marrow and gut. And with both chemotherapy and radiation, there is nausea and diarrhea. Often, you lose your hair and feel constantly weak. So why live?

I decided against those treatments—not because of their side effects but because they affected the entire body adversely, and because I honestly had not seen any of those treatments work. I'd known people who had died after those treatments. Gary had died.

Some of the experimental treatments I'd read about when I was fighting for Gary's life had seemed so logical, experimental or not. Maybe if I'd tried them right away with Gary instead of bullshitting with Dr. Hemp, I could have saved him. Somehow it made more sense to try to get the body on the right track, instead of pumping it full of poisons.

I didn't know exactly what I was going to do when I got home, but I thought I would do some more reading on my disease. When it came time to start treatments, maybe I'd have a head start on the doctors, if I could just gather some strength. Maybe—I actually began to hope—maybe I'd be able to save my life.

# Chapter 12

Dᴀᴠɪᴅ ᴅʀᴏᴠᴇ ᴍᴇ ʜᴏᴍᴇ from the hospital more slowly than he usually drives, taking the dips in the road carefully and easing to his stops so that he wouldn't jostle me.

We came to a red light and he turned to me, his smile surprisingly gentle. "You okay, Mom?"

David had become a handsome teenager—outgoing, dark like his older brothers, with a spontaneous grin and twinkling eyes. It was his gentleness that always surprised me, though. It wasn't like a young kid to be so gentle.

I decided not to answer with my usual lie. I decided to tell him how I felt, but I wasn't thinking about pain at the moment. I was thinking about going home and what I'd find there. The house had probably become a mess in my absence, and it would be filled with David's friends. I'd be greeted by chaos, confusion, and loud noise. So much needed to be done. "David, I can't live another month with those kitchen cupboards the way they are," I said.

He looked at me as if I'd flipped. "What?" he said. "What are you talking about, Mother?"

I started to tell him that I wanted to die in pleasant surroundings, with nice kitchen cupboards, but I knew it wasn't the thing to say. He wasn't even aware of how sick I was. I hadn't wanted to tell him.

Loud music blared from my house as we drove into the driveway. David had left his band rehearsing while he came to pick me up. He helped me out of the car and carried my suitcase into the house, where the harsh rock music was pounding mercilessly. It wasn't so bad when they played rock and roll. David loved the music of the fifties and still imitated Elvis Presley. The fifties act his band put on for parties and weddings went over well. I thought it was great. But this other stuff they sometimes played—this noise—it grated on my nerves.

Mama greeted me at the door, hands over her ears, trying to talk over the music. "Bossie, how you gonna get well with all this racket?"

"Just as long as my kids are healthy, Mama, let them play their music," I said wearily. But she didn't hear me. And I was too weak to scream over the music. I laid my coat and scarf on the sofa and stood in a daze in the middle of the room.

"Bossie, go lie down. I fixed your bed for you. You look tired," said Mama.

"Not right now, Mama. I will in a minute." I searched her face. "Hey, Mama, you look tired yourself. You've been overdoing. You should be the one lying down."

"No, no, Bossie. Here, sit on the couch and rest while I start dinner. I'm making chicken soup."

"Good, Mama." I managed a weak smile. She was the chicken soup mother of the century. Just as I had been.

I stood alone in my living room. There was a banner strung from one side of the room to the other that read "Welcome Home Mom." One end of the banner was sagging a little where the tape had lost its hold, but it was a thoughtful gesture.

My tropical plants were thriving. Mama had taken good care of them during my absence. I walked through the living room and stepped down into the den where the band was practicing. One of the band members—Steve, the short one with the cute blond natural—looked up from his drums. "Hi, Mrs. Wallin, welcome back," he said cheerily.

"Thanks, Steve," I said. But the comfortable, flippant attitude I'd always had around David's friends was completely gone. "Say Steve, you know the music bothers my mother. She's too old for that kind of loud music. Could you guys turn it down, please?"

"Oh sure, Mrs. Wallin."

As I eased myself down into the chair nearest the steps I realized that Mama didn't mind the music so much, it was me. And to Steve I must have looked like Mama's mother that day. I felt like Mama's mother.

But it was good to be home despite the mess and confusion. I leaned back in my chair and just took it all in.

We had a step-down den because it had cost less to build that way. Making it floor level would have meant another truckload of cement, which we could not afford. I had wanted sliding doors so that I could step out into the backyard, but I had settled for two windows.

I knew every corner, every panel, every nail that I had hammered in as I worked alongside the carpenters to save a laborer's pay. I glanced at the spots where the stain was uneven and where there was an inch-long strip of molding missing. I smiled. Proudly. No one but me would ever notice the mistakes. I'd done a terrific job.

Somehow I'd managed to overcome the obstacles and get the den built. It hadn't been easy—negotiating bank loans, looking at blueprints, working side by side with carpenters, running a house, and being a medical typist in the evenings when the kids were asleep.

Since it had been strictly my own idea, I ·didn't mind pitching in. Of course, Jack had objected to the idea of a den. It meant using some of his precious gambling money.

But I ignored his scowls, his sarcastic remarks, and his silent treatments, and I got the den built.

Even the rest of the house looked good. The secondhand furniture—I loved it so much. I'd chosen carefully, bartered, had made sure it was clean before it was delivered. It looked almost elegant to me. No one would take it for secondhand stuff. New furniture would be nice, but I was content with what we had. Yeah . . . it was good to be home.

But the loud music was beginning to get to me. I stood up weakly and went into the kitchen, where Mama was standing over a pot, skimming the fat off the chicken soup. She noticed my worn expression and put down the soup spoon to cup my face in her thin, white hands.

"Bossie, I know what the doctor said about you having cancer again," she said softly. "But you'll be all right, Bossie. Don't cry. You'll be okay."

I wasn't crying, but she knew I was crying inside. And when she said that, tears began to course down my cheeks.

David strolled into the kitchen and stopped short when he saw me crying. "What's wrong, Mom? Is the music too loud?"

"No honey, it's not the music." I bit my lip and wiped the tears away. "I was thinking about the kitchen cupboards," I said like an idiot. "See how awful they are? They stick out like a sore thumb compared to the rest of the house."

He scrutinized the cupboards and said, "Well, what's wrong with them, Mom? What do you want to do with them?"

"Just modernize them, I guess. Look at those hideous things. They're old and beat up. Thick coats of paint one on top of the other. They're terrible. A disgrace. I've wanted to replace them for years and now I'm going to do it."

David looked at me lovingly, then grabbed an apple from the fruit bowl on the kitchen table. "Go lie down,

Mother, you need your rest. You'll get your kitchen cupboards. I know you." He took a giant bite from his apple and then strode back into the den.

Mama stood there, the spoon back in her hand, looking at me as if I were crazy.

"Mama," I said, trying to control the tremor in my voice. "I want to look at pretty things, even if I am going to die."

Mama grabbed me and hugged me and we swayed together in the middle of the kitchen floor.

The three months that followed were considered a waiting period. We were waiting to find out what effects the hysterectomy would have on my cancer. I was waiting to see what effects it would have on my sanity.

For weeks I walked around the house like a zombie, doped up on pain killers and tranquilizers. I had no energy for anything, let alone the research I wanted to do on my disease. The cancer books and magazines in my house remained untouched, and I simply existed for a while.

I had a lot of pain and was so weak I couldn't even wear a wrist watch, because it felt like a grandfather clock on my arm. I had lost thirty pounds and looked like hell.

With the little money we had, I couldn't afford to go any place spectacular. Sometimes I'd go to the market or take short walks in front of the house.

Mama had an arthritis attack about two weeks after I got home and took to her bed in North Hollywood. The house became a mess but I didn't care. We couldn't afford a cleaning woman or a nurse, so I did the best I could. Whenever I was able, I cooked meals and did the dishes. No one else in the house knew how to do those things, so if I didn't do them, we ate at MacDonald's and the dishes piled high in the sink.

I was constantly nauseated. I could barely hold down a bite of food. At times it was just too much effort to raise a fork to my mouth. I felt like a corpse, one in which cancer cells crawled about like fleas on a dog.

Because of the severity of the nausea, I became convinced that the cancer had spread to my stomach. What other reason could there be for feeling so sick?

One day, in a fit of paranoiac depression, I asked David to call Dr. Eisen for me. "Honey, tell the doctor I'm so nauseated I can't eat a thing. See what he says, David. Please."

"So what could it be, Mom? You just got out of the hospital a few days ago. Naturally . . ."

I laughed. "A few days, huh? Ha! David, it's been three weeks. Now go call Dr. Eisen. Something's wrong, and I just don't feel like getting on the phone."

He wasn't convinced. "Look, don't worry about it, Mother. It's probably just . . ."

"David, something is wrong," I insisted.

"Like what?"

"Like, maybe it's spread already."

"What's spread?"

"The cancer, David."

"Mom, you don't . . ." His face turned ashen. "You don't have cancer again, do you, Mom?"

I nodded.

"You didn't tell me."

"I didn't want you to know."

He sat down. Or I should say he fell into a chair, as if he'd been slugged. But he was clearly annoyed with me.

"Why not?" he demanded.

"I just didn't."

"So how bad is it this time?"

"Bad," I told him. "And I think it's hit my stomach, David. I'm so sick I can hardly stand it. Please, honey. Go talk to Dr. Eisen. See what he says. Would you do that for me?"

He did as I asked and then came back to report to me. "Look Mom, he says the reason you feel so weak and nauseous is because of what you've been through, that's all—the loss of blood and being in surgery for six hours. And the nausea is caused by all the medications you got at the hospital."

"David, I'm sorry," I said wearily. "I just didn't want you to know."

Then I started to cry. My son did, too. He hugged me. "It's okay, Mom. Hey. It's really okay."

Mechanically and in constant pain, I tried to tend to the household chores, resenting the fact that I got no help from anyone, but unwilling to ask for help. It wasn't that David was a bum. He was very helpful in trying to lift my spirits. But he never thought to wash the dishes or vacuum the rug or do the laundry because I'd spoiled my kids rotten all their lives. I had never let them lift a finger when they were growing up.

David never took on any of the household chores, but one day he came home from school with a cane he'd rented from some orthopedic store for me. A cane! Not a bad-looking one, but a cane! I cracked up.

David pointed out practically that I needed one. And I did. He was a thoughtful kid for seventeen.

Sometimes, when I wanted to get out of the house, I'd get in my car and take little joy rides. David went on one of those joy rides. He was looking around for a second-hand guitar. One afternoon he came to me and said, "Mom, I found a great guitar. I can't decide whether or not to buy it. It's a little more than I was planning to spend and I don't know if it's worth it. Will you go with me now to look at it?"

It sounded like fun, so I went. I took another pain pill before we left and things were quite fuzzy. I wasn't thinking clearly enough to ask David to drive, so I got in behind the wheel. I am ashamed now to think that I endangered his life, but I wasn't in the habit of thinking about my safety. If I was going to die, I actually preferred a head-on collision to cancer.

We got onto the freeway and I began weaving along, zipping in and out of lanes, until David gasped and said, "Jeez, Mom, don't kill us!"

By the time we got to the music store, David was a wreck. "From now on, I'm driving," he said. "Mom, you could really kill yourself driving like that. From now on, when you want to go somewhere, let me know and I'll drive you." And the kid worked his college schedule around so he could drive me to most of the places I wanted to go.

One day when he wasn't around, I sneaked off to the drugstore to fill a prescription for Darvon and backed right into a woman's car. Not surprising. I wasn't looking where I was going and probably wouldn't have seen it had I looked. My insurance company fixed the damage and my insurance rates went up.

Having David around those days helped to take my mind off the terror. One night, very late, I was sitting alone in the house in my rocking chair watching television. David had gone out on a date and Jack hadn't come home from Gardena yet. I sat there staring at the television set. The pain pulsed rhythmically in time to my rocking.

Finally David threw open the front door and stomped into the den, tossing his keys onto the sofa. He sank there, browsing in the *TV Guide*.

"H'lo, Mom," he muttered. He flipped through the pages as if he were going to tear them out and eat them any minute.

"What's the matter, David?"

He glanced up briefly. "Oh, nothing," he said and went back to his *TV Guide*.

"Nothing, huh? You act like you just got punched out. Did Pam punch you out tonight?"

He didn't laugh.

"So what is it? Did you and Pam disagree?"

"Oh no. Uh-uh, we didn't disagree," he snapped. "We just broke up, that's all."

I rocked back and forth quietly. Sometimes it pays to shut up. It brings the words faster than anything else.

"Aw, who gives a shit anyway?" he mumbled.

"Well, obviously you do," I replied.

"Women," he spluttered. "They're impossible to understand. You know what she said? She said I was getting too heavy."

"I told you not to eat so many of those candy bars," I joked.

"Very funny," he said, making a face at me. "Heavy, Mom. Too serious or something."

"Were you?"

He thought for a minute. "Yeah, I guess I was. I really liked her. I thought everything was going great, too. We were going up to Big Bear Friday and everything, and we had plans to go down to Newport over Christmas vacation to visit her folks. Now all of a sudden she wants to see other guys. Okay. Fine with me. I should care." His voice had reached a fervent pitch. He looked ready to hurl the *TV Guide* in my face.

"Come here, David."

"What for?" he asked me sullenly, pushing his nose into the guide. He was pouting.

"Just come here," I said.

Reluctantly he got up and dragged his feet all the way to my chair. He sat down at my feet, crossed his legs and looked up at me.

"So big deal," I told him. "So you'll get another girlfriend. You're just mad because you got rejected."

He looked down at the floor. "No, I'm mad because she's such a phony."

"Now, David. Think about it. It got to your ego, didn't it?"

He sighed. "Yeah. Okay. I guess it did."

"Well, it's not the first time you've been rejected and it won't be the last," I told him. "So you'll call that girl I heard you telling Steve about the other day."

A smile tugged at the corners of his mouth. "What girl?" he asked me innocently.

"The one with the big boobs," I said triumphantly.

He rolled back his eyes, clapped his hands to his forehead, and laughed. "Okay, okay!" he said. "What do you do, listen in on all my conversations or only some of them?"

"Some of them."

He shook his head at me. "You're right," he said, patting my knee softly. "I'll get over it. Like you said, so what's the big deal? Life goes on."

The problem resolved, he turned back to the television and became instantly engrossed in some John Wayne movie. He'd figured out that night what was taking me years to discover—life goes on.

But if life was going to go on, I was determined to get my kitchen cupboards renovated. I still wasn't prepared to delve into the cancer material lying around my house. It would be an enormous project, and the thought of going back into the gruesome details of my disease depressed me.

But I wanted to be involved in something worthwhile, so the next morning, when I heard the water going in the bathroom and knew Jack was getting ready for work, I knocked on the bathroom door.

"Jack. Jack, I want to talk to you," I called in to him.

He opened the door. He was shaving. "What is it, Bernice?"

"I want to talk to you about the kitchen cupboards. I'm getting new doors put on them," I informed him.

Jack didn't miss a stroke, but I saw a frown appear beneath the shaving cream. "Kitchen cupboards? How are you going to manage that with all the doctor bills?" he asked me calmly.

My defense flared. "Why is it always how I'm going to manage these things?"

"Well, I've got expenses of my own!"

"You call gambling *expenses?*"

"Hey, the kitchen looks fine," he tried to humor me.

"Everything looks fine to you. If the ceiling fell in, you'd say it looked fine."

"Why do you have to have them redone right now? Why not wait a while?"

"Because I need them now. Now that I'm going to be home all day, I want a nice kitchen to look at while I'm dying."

He cringed. "So get 'em," he said and closed the door in my face.

But as usual, Jack's attitude was enough to quell my enthusiasm.

And then my guilt popped up. Do I ask for too much? Am I trying to live beyond my means? Maybe I'm being a prima donna. How badly do I really want the kitchen cupboards? Am I being ridiculous? And how long would I get to enjoy them anyway?

There was no question in my mind that they were genuinely important to me. The length of time I had them was not the issue. And I didn't care what the rest of the family thought, either. But there was more to it than that, I realized. There was some sort of superstition involved. As if by investing in something as trivial as kitchen cabinets, I might get to hang around a little longer. And, of course, it would give me a reason to get out of bed in the morning. And that in itself was something. It was enough for starters.

So that was it. I was going to get the cupboards.

A few days later I picked up a Culver City newspaper at a newsstand and leafed through the pages to the classified section. My eyes skimmed the page. I knew exactly what I was looking for—someone who didn't charge too much. And there it was, an ad that said something about a retired carpenter who considered no job too big or too small and whose fees were reasonable.

For days we were surrounded by the chaos of boxes, tools, and paint cans. The loud hammering and sawing was music to my ears. It brought back the days of the den-building. And in very short order, I had new cupboard doors. Bright, shiny, and modern.

But after they were finished and I'd packed everything neatly away, I was ready for more. I wanted wallpaper, colorful wallpaper. And maybe a new stove. Not really new, maybe just a little newer than the one I had. I'd sell the old stove and with that money I'd buy one of those frost-free refrigerators. Thoughts like these didn't ease my physical pain, but they sure helped lighten my spirit.

One day I stopped at a paint store and selected the wallpaper and all the things I needed to redo my kitchen walls.

David came home from school to find me standing on the kitchen table doing my best to apply the wallpaper. I had taken some pills and was royally stoned. I must have been weaving a little, because David gasped and said, "Mom, what the hell are you doing? You're going to kill yourself up there."

"No I'm not, I'm going to die from cancer, remember?" I said cheerily. "At least I'll have a nice kitchen to do it in, and when your father remarries, his wife will be able to cook your dinners in a nice kitchen. Right?"

"Oh stop it," David said. "You're not going to die." He grabbed my hand to pull me off the table.

"We're all going to die some day. Now leave me be, David. There's work to do."

And a damn good job I did, too. The wallpaper and cupboard doors cost me only $440. And I loved them as much as if they'd cost $40,000.

# Chapter 13

I HAD FREQUENT APPOINTMENTS with Dr. Eisen and my surgeon during this waiting period, but there seemed to be nothing either of them could tell me.

"We're playing the waiting game," Dr. Eisen chuckled one day, trying to put me in a good humor, I guess.

"You're making jokes with my life," I told him grimly. The lady with zilch sense of humor.

When the smile left his face, I felt satisfied. I was losing patience with all doctors, even my beloved Dr. Eisen.

"I'm not making jokes, Bernice, we . . ."

"You what? You keep saying 'we.' 'We're' waiting for this, 'we' don't know that. Who is this royal 'we?' It's *me*. I'm the one who's waiting. You don't know what waiting is, Dr. Eisen. For you, waiting is sitting here at your desk waiting for a lab report to come back. For me, waiting is sitting around my house wondering if I'm going to die. I just want you to tell me how long I've got, and I want you to tell me straight."

Sometimes he looked as if he wanted to strike me. As if it were all he could do to keep from screaming at me. He waited a minute, played with a pencil on his desk, and then he tried to respond to my outburst with his marvelous self-control.

"We—and I do mean *we*, Bernice, because believe it or not I'm with you on this thing all the way—we are waiting to see what the results of the hysterectomy will be. Response is not always favorable. It takes about two months for estrogen to leave the body, which may alleviate the pain. It doesn't mean the cancer will leave, just the pain. But Bernice, please, we have to wait and see."

Those appointments were always accompanied by a thumping session. He'd thump me all over, asking me if it hurt, feeling under my ribs for my spleen and liver, probing my armpits and around the neck area back under my ears, looking for lymph nodes. If there were nodes, they'd have to operate immediately.

When I got home from those sessions, I would check for nodes myself, around my neck and under my arms. I did that for hours, until I was beet red and sore all over. If I thought I felt a node, I would fall apart completely. I wouldn't be able to wash a dish or eat. I couldn't watch television, listen to the radio or anything. I could only lie in bed, trembling, until the next doctor's visit, when he could tell me if the malignancy had spread to the lymph nodes. Once it does that, you're practically gone. You can count your days.

One evening as I lay in my bed after one of these private thumping sessions, Jack poked his head in the door of the bedroom. "I was just on my way out to pick up a hamburger. Want one?"

"Yes I do," I replied. "If you can remember after twenty-five years of marriage that I don't like relish or onions on my hamburger."

He simply closed the door quietly.

I hated myself for acting that way. And after he'd closed the door, I realized it was time to stop lying around playing Camille. To spend all the remaining hours of my life in bed or sitting around probing myself, to yell at my family and play the martyr, well, it just made no sense.

I began to face reality. I started being more active. I quit picking on Jack and started trying to be more amiable.

By the first of October, the pain was beginning to diminish. By late October, there was almost no pain. Instead of taking pain killers every two hours, I cut them down to every four hours, and soon I needed them only every six hours.

At first I didn't notice I was taking pills less often, until one day I noticed the bottle of pain killers was still almost full. That's when I realized I'd been walking around in a cloud for the last several weeks, almost completely out of touch with my physical self, except for the pain. When I saw the number of pills left, I started to become conscious of my body again, and when I did, I also realized there wasn't as much pain. I felt freer, almost normal.

I began to do the things I had always loved doing. I went to the library and to museums. I felt like someone released from a concentration camp.

One day I dressed for autumn, grabbing a bag of sunflower seeds and a coat and heading for the Marina in my car. I parked and got out to walk. It was a little past noon. The sun was shining. It was crisp and exhilarating outside. There was a refreshing breeze from the ocean which perked up my spirits.

I walked along the wharf and watched the boats. I felt the sun on my·back and welcomed the wind on my face. I felt good.

The light glinted on the water like bits of broken glass and the boats bobbed merrily up and down. I entered the bird sanctuary at the end of the wharf. There was no one else around. I hummed an old favorite tune and tossed handfuls of seeds to the ducks. I felt like a little girl again. I thought about Papa, about how nice it had been to be protected as a child.

In a few minutes, I was surrounded by birds. As I walked, they followed me. I felt like a queen followed by a comic entourage.

I was going to do this more often, I told myself. Why not every day! Life was so beautiful, I informed myself. "How could you ever have been so miserable, Bernice?"

That night I could hardly wait until Jack got home. I was going to ask him to take me dancing. The way we used to years ago. Besides, the years were beginning to catch up with Jack. Even his holy pilgrimages to Gardena were less frequent. He just might find time.

My heart leaped when I heard him pull into the driveway. He had hardly stepped one foot in the house when I attacked. "Hey Jack," I said. I felt like a mischievous little kid. "Let's go dancing tonight. What do you say?"

He acted as if I had told him a very funny story. He laughed heartily, patted me on the back, and then made his way to the den, where his old friend the television was waiting for him. I followed him.

"No, I'm serious, Jack. I feel good. C'mon, remember when we used to go dancing? When we were young?"

"We're not young any more, Bernice," he told me. "Besides, you're sick. You need to rest."

"I've been resting for two months, Jack," I insisted. "C'mon, we'll go out to dinner, then we'll stop at the Trolley Car in Santa Monica. They've got a nice big dance floor there. What's the matter? You too old? You forget how to dance?"

"I'll take you out to dinner, sure. But I'm tired, Bernice, you forget, I work all day. You're crazy. Dancing. At our age."

"At our age? What are we? A hundred years old or something?"

But he would have none of it. We went out to dinner,

came home early.. And he went promptly to bed. But oh, how I wanted to go dancing. I sat in my rocking chair in the den that night and remembered what it was like to dance, how my shoulder-length hair would fly around when I swayed to the music. It was a glorious feeling, almost like a swimming sensation in my head. The music had seemed to lift me to the clouds. I'd always thought dancing represented a rebellious spirit—an independent spirit. And how good I'd been once. Jack was a fairly good dancer too. Once. A long, long time ago.

November passed quickly. In the back of my mind was that reading I wanted to do on cancer treatments, but I was enjoying the pain-free period so much, I decided to wait. Not having any pain was such a luxury.

When Thanksgiving came, I felt almost like myself, before the pain had ever started. I felt good enough to roast a turkey and have the family over to celebrate. Paul and Sharon came and Jack's two sisters and their husbands. Fred was still working in Boston and couldn't be there, but David was there. All in all, I was pretty grateful about everything.

By December I was feeling anxious about what Dr. Eisen was going to recommend in the way of treatment. I knew that soon he would try to put me on drugs or suggest radiation or more surgery.

At one of my checkups, I said to him, "Okay, doctor, so you told me we were waiting for the results of the hysterectomy. So what are the results?"

"Well, Bernice, we know that the hysterectomy relieved the pain. And to tell you the truth," he went on, "I just don't know what to do with you. We just have to wait. That's all."

"Wait?" Surely he wasn't going to wait 'till I died to start discussing treatment with me. "How much longer?"

"Well, we've accomplished the first order of business. We've removed the ovaries," he said. "Now we can try chemotherapy pretty soon. And with chemotherapy . . ."

"I know about chemotherapy, Dr. Eisen, and you can forget it," I said.

He looked mildly annoyed. "Now Bernice," he said, "chemotherapy is one of the recognized treatments for a metastasis. So it must have some merits."

I shook my head silently.

He was exasperated. "What is wrong with this woman?" his eyes seemed to say. "Now there's an adrenalectomy, the removal of the adrenal glands, which also cuts down on the estrogen and sometimes . . ."

"Look, I don't want to hear any more of this, Dr. Eisen," I told him. "You know how I feel about traditional cancer treatments. They don't work. I don't want my brain cut out. I don't want my adrenal glands removed. And I don't want anyone to beam radiation at my oh-so-few healthy cells."

"What do you want from me, Bernice? A miracle? I've told you what we can do, and you don't want to do any of it. So now what?"

So now, I told myself, it was time. It was time to start going to other doctors. Eisen was no specialist. He knew three words when it came to cancer treatment: chemotherapy, radiation, and surgery. I'd go talk to some oncologists. I'd find out what was happening in the cancer field.

That day I left Dr. Eisen's office thinking about fighting my disease. I didn't want to be half a person while I was alive. I'd rather be dead.

I drove home from Dr. Eisen's office in a state of confusion, my mind racing with thoughts like so many wild horses.

I fixed dinner in that state, shaking spices all over a chicken and popping it with potatoes into the oven.

And then in the middle of all this emotional turmoil, David burst into the house like a wild Indian. "Mom! Mom! We got the gig! We got it!"

"The gig, honey? What gig?"

"At the Classic Cat!" he cried, jumping up and down like a five-year-old. "Yippee!"

Yippee wasn't quite how I felt about this gig or any-thing else at the moment. The Classic Cat was a strip joint in Hollywood on Sunset Boulevard. I considered it a sleazy joint. David and his band had auditioned for a one-night job there a week before.

"But, honey, why almost at the last minute do they call you?" I said, but I couldn't help smiling at him hopping across the floor.

"Well, the man explained that the other band backed out and would we please fill in. Hey, I don't care if we're second choice! We're going to play! We're going to get paid! Yippee!"

He'd been paid for entertaining before, but this was his first night club job. So, despite my jumbled state of mind, my wondering about what I was going to do to stay alive, Jack and I went to the Classic Cat.

Of all the places to go when you're riddled with cancer, the Classic Cat seems like the last place. Dancing at a nice place with a big dance floor and an orchestra or dance band would have been fine. But to watch a bunch of people smoking, drinking, and taking off their clothes—it was crazy. But I went there to see David, so it didn't matter what anyone else was doing.

When they introduced David's band, it was one of the thrills of my life. A smile grew and grew on my face until it was all I could do to keep from jumping up and hugging him. Everyone in the joint must have known that I was the mother of someone up there. I hoped that they wouldn't think it was one of the half-nude girls on stage with my son.

David did the Elvis routine I loved so much. He wore the tight trousers with silver studs and the white floor-length cape with fringe I'd sewn for him a year earlier.

He enjoyed himself on stage and didn't even seem to notice the two naked girls with enormous fans on either side of him. He was so cool, so sophisticated, up there carrying on with his life.

And that's what I was going to do, too, I told myself. I

was going to get on with my life. First thing in the morning, I was going to call another doctor. Since when was Dr. Eisen God? He was a *mench vee alleh menchen,* a man like all men. There were different ways of doing things, and I was going to find a way that would work for me.

But the morning after David's performance at the Classic Cat, I woke up with a sharp pain in my leg. It was the first time I'd felt pain in weeks, and it was in my leg again. It felt like a million arrows were piercing my body.

*It's still there,* I thought. *It's eating away at my insides.*

Then I tried to rationalize my fear. And I used the same stupid rationalizations I'd used the first time the pain showed up in my leg. Rheumatism, a touch of arthritis, just a bad day.

But it didn't go away. I had to start coping with that damned excruciating pain all over again. Thoughts of fighting for my life left me, and I just went around the house mechanically doing chores again.

I called Dr. Eisen and tried to talk it over with him— told him the pain was killing me. All he said was, "Let's wait. Just a little while longer."

I felt as if my body were being sliced with a knife. It was too much to bear. I had to talk to someone about it. I couldn't talk to David. I didn't want to worry him. Maybe I should see a psychiatrist. After all, it was not only my body that was tortured. My mind was in agony, too.

But damn it, why should I have to see a shrink? I had a husband. I'd beg if I had to. I'd plead with Jack to talk to me, to listen to me, to respond—just this once.

He came home from work in a pretty good humor the day I'd planned to talk it over with him.

"Hi honey, brought some cookies," he said, striding through the kitchen and throwing two packages on the kitchen table.

"Did you have a good day?" I started brightly.

"It was all right. What's for dinner?" He walked past

me into the den and plopped himself down in front of the television set.

"Beef stew," I said, following him slowly. "Jack, would you mind turning off the set for a few minutes? I'd like to talk to you."

He lowered the sound on the set, but his eyes remained glued to the screen. I started talking about trivia at first. Wanted to test him, to throw out a piece of bait and see if he'd go for it. "Got a letter from Fred today," I said. I studied his face to see if this sparked any interest.

"You did? What does he write?"

"Says he's doing great. Making pretty good money. Says he may be home this summer to visit."

"Mmm-hmmm."

Then I started rambling about David's new guitar, his schoolwork, about Mama and how she was doing. Finally I worked up enough nerve to talk about myself. I told him that I wasn't feeling well, that the pain in my leg had returned. That it was bad.

"What do you think, Jack? Dr. Eisen tells me that even though the pain is back, I should keep it in check with pain killers and wait and see. I ask him how long I should wait and he says he doesn't know. I ask if he has treated other women with the same condition, and he's vague about it. I ask him if he can show me anyone with a metastasis who has lived any length of time after the removal of the ovaries, and he's still vague. He's so vague, Jack. I don't know what to do. He talks more surgery, chemotherapy. I just don't know. What do you think?"

"Bernice. Why are you asking me? How the hell would I know? You're the one who knows all about cancer. Not me. Go ask the doctor."

The hurt surged in my throat. "Jack, I need someone to help me decide what to do. It's too much for one person to have to cope with this."

"What can I tell you? What do you want me to say?"

"How about a few words of comfort, Jack? How about

a few of those? Like how about trying to help me figure out what to do with the so-called rest of my life?"

Actually I didn't know what it was exactly I wanted from him. If only he'd tried to talk about it, I think that would have been enough.

"You're my husband," I said. "And when I talk to you about my life, you watch television. You listen to the women at the butcher shop tell you their troubles. That's what you tell me. Why can't you do the same for me? You're . . . you're . . ." I left the room in tears. I felt like someone who had been caught talking to a tree in the park.

I went back to the kitchen and turned the flame on under the pot of beef stew. My thoughts began racing madly in my head, like a hamster on a wheel. Round and round they went as I stared into space, cooking dinner, stirring the stew, cooking dinner, stirring the stew. Gary, my lousy marriage, my pain. Jack was about as sympathetic as a concrete sidewalk. That's all there was to it. It's your life, Bernice, not his, I told myself bitterly. He has no stake in your life. His stakes are all in Gardena.

The next few days were gray and dismal and cold. All I could think about was my pain. I sat in my rocking chair in the den and stared into space most of the day. Fight this thing? Ha! It was just too much trouble. Sometimes I wondered if living was worth the effort anyway.

# Chapter 14

DECEMBER WORE ON, each day like a year.

Then came the turning point in my life. It was some time in December. I can't remember the exact day. If I could remember the date, I'd celebrate it every year with firecrackers and hundreds of bright colored balloons.

I was standing in line at the checkout counter in the market, my body wracked with pain, when my eye caught the headline on a *National Enquirer:* "New Vaccine Battles Cancer."

The *National Enquirer* was not the kind of newspaper I usually read, but naturally the headline intrigued me. I picked up the paper and flipped back to the article. It looked very interesting. I tossed it into my cart.

By the time I got out to my car in the parking lot, hope was racing through me. A new cure, huh? A new approach?

I piled the groceries into the front seat and hurriedly

pulled out the newspaper. The article stated that there was a UCLA doctor giving a vaccine called Bacillus Calmette Guerin, or BCG, to build up a person's immunity against cancer.

Immunity. That approach was familiar to me. I'd read a few things about the immune system when Gary was sick. We had tried one therapy in which cancer cells from Gary's own urine had been injected to activate his immune system.

And I remembered that Dr. William Dameshek, a Boston physician, had told me with such conviction that leukemia was caused by a malfunctioning immune system.

That's what the *National Inquirer* article was saying—that the immune system might have some relationship to cancer control.

I felt strangely excited. I drove all the way home with a big grin on my face.

I tossed the groceries in their proper places, poured myself a glass of apple juice, popped a few pain pills, and called Dr. Eisen.

The nurse told me he was busy with a patient.

I told her to have him call me when he could spare a few minutes.

"What's wrong, Mrs. Wallin? Is anything wrong?" she asked kindly.

"No, no, but just have him call me. I want to talk to him the minute he is free," I replied.

I set about preparing dinner, humming to myself. While I was grating carrots, Dr. Eisen returned my call.

"What's up, Bernice? Nancy says you sounded excited. Is anything wrong?"

"No, but I think I've just run across something that may save my life."

"You have, huh? What have you run across, Bernice? Tell me about it."

"Do you know anything about BCG, doctor?"

He paused. "Well, I know BCG was discovered in the

early 1900s by two French doctors—Albert Calmette and Camille Guerin. I know that it was used in this country as an anti-TB vaccine in the twenties. It hasn't been used much since. Only in Europe."

"Do you know anything about its relationship to cancer?"

"To cancer? No. What are you talking about, Bernice?"

"Doctor, I have an article in my hand that I've cut out of the *National Enquirer* that tells about BCG's being given to cancer patients. And it's showing good results."

"Listen, Bernice, if it's in one of those newspapers, you might as well forget it."

"Why? Because it came out of a certain newspaper you don't like? It says here—listen, let me read it to you: 'A vaccination that can protect all mankind against getting cancer is possible within the next twenty years, says one of the nation's leading cancer researchers. The vaccination, he says, will involve the amazing BCG vaccine.' Then it goes on to say that this doctor is giving the vaccine, and he thinks it works."

There was silence on Dr. Eisen's end of the line. "Doctor? Are you there?"

"Bernice, I wouldn't trust anything out of a paper like that," he said.

"You mean what it says here about experiments being conducted with this vaccine—that's not true?"

"Who knows, Bernice, those papers are just a bunch of sensational garbage. And just because they're experimenting doesn't mean you can get it. Where are they giving this vaccine?"

I was annoyed. "It doesn't say exactly in the article, but I'm going to check on it," I said.

"Suit yourself, Bernice," he replied.

I called UCLA to find out whether or not they were doing the BCG experiments at their clinic, and the reply was affirmative.

Now the spark was ignited. I was excited as hell. I

called Jack at work that evening and told him I'd leave dinner in the refrigerator for him.

"Where are you off to at dinnertime?" he asked.

"The library, Jack, and it's very important, so don't go getting all upset. There's a chicken in the refrigerator and a salad. If you want a potato, throw it in the oven when you get home."

It wasn't at all like me to do that sort of thing, and I guess I felt pretty guilty as I grabbed my jacket and jumped into the car. But the man was an adult. He could put the food on the table himself.

I got on the freeway and headed for the UCLA biomedical library. I'd been there so many times when Gary was sick, the car practically drove itself.

I was racing to the library as if my life depended on it. I felt my life did depend on it. But when I saw a blinking red light in my rear view mirror, I knew I was driving much too fast.

I pulled over and watched in my mirror as the officer got out of his car and sauntered to my window.

"What's the hurry, ma'am?" he asked me.

"Doctor . . . I mean, I mean 'officer,' I. . . . " I was stuttering like a fool.

He looked at me strangely and poked his head into my car. "Have you been drinking?" he wanted to know.

I wasn't even high on pain killers at the moment. My head was spinning from all the adrenalin pumping through my veins. He was pulling out his citation book.

"Officer, please listen," I begged. I reached into my purse and pulled out the newspaper clipping I'd cut from the paper. "Please read this." I handed him the clipping, explaining wildly, "Look, I have cancer. I just read this article and I was on my way to the biomedical library at UCLA to get more information on it. I'm thinking maybe it can help me. I'm sorry I was speeding, but I just got so excited about the article. And I may not have much time to live as it is. I guess I was just trying to save a few extra minutes."

He took out his flashlight, squinted at the article, and perused its contents. Then he smiled at me compassionately. "Well, just be careful," he said. "You wouldn't want to have an accident just when you're getting ready to save your own life, now would you?"

"You mean you're not going to give me a ticket?"

He folded the article and handed it to me. "Just drive a little slower," he said, and walked back to his patrol car.

So thank goodness, no ticket. I started my car again and didn't slow down in the least. I sped into the parking lot off Westwood Boulevard. It was crammed with cars, as usual. I parked, took my cane, hobbled toward the campus. Walking around UCLA always confused me. It was so huge. It's more than just a university with ivory towers of learning. There's quite a hospital there, too—complete medical facilities, clinics with services from pediatrics to psychiatric care.

The campus had changed a lot since the last time I was there, seven years earlier. There were new buildings. Windows bricked over. New entrances, new gates, new signs. But somehow I found the library and managed to grope my way past the turnstyle with my cane.

Just the smell of the books excited me. Books have a marvelous aroma. I wasn't panic-stricken that evening, as I'd been when I went there to do research on leukemia.

I found the huge computer printout books and flipped to the I's for immunotherapy . . . not much there. Then, for the sake of curiosity, I went ahead to the L's and looked up leukemia. And what research had been done since I'd last scanned those pages! When Gary was sick, there had been about a third of what I found that night. I was glad to know that other kids might have a better chance than my son.

I went back to the entry for immunotherapy and wrote down the names of some books. Then I wandered through the stacks until I found some of the ones on my list. I picked a few and then sat down in a cozy niche to read.

It was so confusing, all those medical terms, the complicated jargon. I must have sat for hours, browsing through books on the latest research, the newest gains made against my disease. For about three hours I read. I read until my head ached and I realized that indeed I'd just given my brain a workout.

I spent a fortune in nickels copying pages from those books, and I left the library feeling invigorated. The pain in my leg didn't seem half as intense as it had that morning.

As I was making my way back to the car, I heard someone call my name.

"Bernice! Bernice Wallin!" A young woman was approaching me, and I recognized Jean Williams, the nurse who had so lovingly cared for Gary. I had come to know her quite well during Gary's last days, and she had called me several times after his death to comfort me and to find out how I was.

She looked as pretty as ever—shiny red hair, clear complexion, clear blue eyes. Ah, yes, the picture of health.

"What is this, Bernice?" she asked, eyeing my cane.

I didn't like telling people about my illness, but she was an old friend and I didn't see any point in lying to her. I told her as simply as I could about what had taken place since Gary's death.

Her eyes were wide as I related the story. We walked toward the parking lot together. "Oh Bernice, I hate to hear all this," she said sympathetically, putting her arm around my shoulders.

"What about you, Jean? What are you doing over here?"

"I'm working here now," she said. "Just got off. Hey, let's go get some coffee. Do you feel like doing that? Really, you look pretty good, Bernice, I . . ."

"Hey, I know how I look, I look like hell," I said with a laugh. "But I'll tell you something, Jean, I feel pretty good tonight. Let's do go have some coffee."

So we sat down together at a local coffee shop and

exchanged more news. Actually I was bursting to tell her about my discovery.

"You have a little gleam in your eye tonight, Bernice," Jean observed. "What's up?"

"Do I really?" I laughed. "Boy. I must really feel hopeful. I didn't know it showed."

"What are you hopeful about?"

I pulled out the article and showed it to her. We sat side by side, reading it silently.

When she'd finished, she looked at me solemnly and ran her hand through her thick, red hair. "What kind of breast cancer did you say you had, Bernice?"

"Carcinoma," I said.

"Well, Bernice, you know, don't you, that carcinoma is quite a different thing from melanoma?"

"Melanoma? Who said anything about melanoma?"

She pointed to the very last paragraph of the article. "It says here . . . let's see . . . it says they're treating melanoma patients with this new vaccine. It doesn't say anything about carcinoma."

"Where?" I said, searching the paragraph. "Where does . . . it say . . . oh yes, here, I see what you mean." That's what it said, all right. I hadn't even seen that sentence. How could I have missed it? I bit my lip and looked out the window.

"Oh, Bernice," she said. "I haven't spoiled your hope, have I?"

It almost came crashing down on my head, the hope. But somehow I managed to keep it from exploding into little fragments, and I said, "You know, Jean, I went right by that sentence and didn't even see it."

"Oh, Bernice."

"But I'm not sure it makes any difference. I mean, I don't know. Who knows? Maybe they're using it on carcinoma patients, too. I'll just have to find out more about it, that's all."

I folded up the article and slipped it back into my purse,

changing the subject. I figured I'd think about it later. I'd just sort it all out later.

And by midnight that night, as I sat poring over the articles on my kitchen table, I was sure it didn't matter. Regardless of what they were doing at UCLA, immunotherapy might offer hope, even if I couldn't understand it completely.

As I kept reading the papers over and over at my kitchen table, I realized that I didn't have enough background to absorb all the information I was trying to cram into my head. The over-all picture would be fascinating, I told myself, if I could just comprehend it.

The pages spoke of cells: B-cells, T-cells, leukocytes. With Gary's leukemia, I had learned how important leukocytes were in fighting infection. I knew that blood was formed in the bone marrow. But I really didn't know enough to understand what I was reading.

I decided that night to run over to the local library the next day and get some basic books on physiology. Before I could understand immunotherapy, I had to understand the basics.

The next day I practically bounced out of bed. Made the beds, did some dishes, grabbed a bite to eat, and I was off for the library. I checked out a couple of college physiology books and sped back home with them.

It was a crisp, clear day, and I decided to read outside. I put on a sweater and some sunglasses and pulled out the rusty old lounge chair that had been in our backyard since day one. I wondered if anyone had ever sat in it to enjoy the sunshine. The kids used to play on it, and it was falling apart. But I threw a blanket over it and decided the sun would do me good.

I started from the beginning.

Cells. Those tiny things so small it would take seven or eight hundred of them to cover a pin. Miniscule living organisms that multiply and specialize to form tissues and organs—the whole human body is made of these crazy little cells. Their growth and division is controlled precisely by biological signals that scientists are only now beginning to understand.

I read until the sun began to go down, and I didn't even look up until a gust of wind blew the pages around. I closed the book. My fingers were numb. I shivered. It was cold.

I ran into the house and saw that I had about ten minutes before Jack got home.

I pulled some hamburger from the refrigerator and started slapping some patties together, my mind still on those beautifully regulated cells that grow and stop in response to mysterious signals in the body.

Except some of mine hadn't stopped when they were supposed to. Maybe they were waiting to be told. "Stop!" I said out loud and laughed. "Stop growing, you stupid cells!"

"What are you doing, Mom, talking to yourself?" asked David, coming up behind me and kissing me on the cheek.

"Just talking to my cells," I said. "Listen, son, did you take out the trash this morning? I didn't look."

"Oh Mom, I forgot all about it," he said. "When's dinner? I'm starved."

I stopped making the patties and just looked at him. "You didn't take out the trash?"

"I forgot," he repeated meekly.

"You forgot. Well, that's nice, David, the trash man doesn't come around again for another week."

He was quiet a few minutes as I continued to prepare dinner. Finally, he said rather sullenly, "Mom. So what's the big deal about the trash?"

"Nothing's a big deal about it, David, I just . . ."

"Well, you always make me feel like I'm a bad person or something, just because I don't take out the trash. You make me feel guilty over such a little thing like that. It's really stupid." He was sitting at the kitchen table, pouting.

I couldn't believe my ears. "David Wallin, I ask you to

do so little around here it's ridiculous. Yes. Yes, you should feel guilty when you can't even do a little thing like taking out the trash. Damn it. Now next week you take it out."

"Don't worry, Mother," he said sarcastically, leaving the kitchen in a huff.

Never had I been so harsh with David over something like that. Usually I just went and did it myself on Thursday mornings if I saw he'd forgotten. Which he usually did. I'd remind him later in the evening, but I'd never reprimanded him. As a matter of fact, I always felt a little guilty about asking him to do it in the first place. You're crazy, Bernice, I told myself. The people in this house aren't your masters. It's a cooperative household, dummy!

But still I felt a little guilty about making David feel guilty. I sighed. Would it never end, this guilt? Would I ever be able to liberate myself and my family from my incessant guilt?

Nevertheless, I was gaining a certain independence from all the research I'd been doing. For once I felt that I had control over my life. And why should trash and dinner and marketing and laundry get in my way? Those were the trivialities in life. They were very unimportant, actually.

But as I delved really deep into my study of cancer, I started feeling another kind of guilt. Why hadn't I devoted this much time to research when Gary was sick? The reading had all been superficial when he was dying. I'd gone from one thing to another, explored one area, then jumped to something else. I never got a total picture— only bits and pieces.

I'd been terrified as I searched for answers to Gary's disease. I got mixed up trying to figure out whether to listen to Hemp, Rosenfeld, Eisen, or one of the hundreds of other doctors I talked to. I'd also had three sons to raise, a house to keep, and a disinterested husband who was never home to help.

Well, history didn't have to repeat itself. I'd done my

best for Gary. This time I had a head start.

But I suddenly realized that I had started learning everything I knew during Gary's illness and after he died. More than that, it was as a result of Gary's dying that I knew as much as I did. The thought made me physically ill. I saw a connection between Gary's dying and my continuing to live—as if Gary had been sacrificed for me. Of course I was jumping the gun. I hadn't been granted BCG yet, and even if I was, I didn't know for sure that it would work. But the thought ate at me just the same, and the guilt was overwhelming.

Why couldn't it have been the other way around? Why couldn't I have been sacrificed so that Gary could have lived? I had had a chance at a life. Gary never had.

But my death could not bring Gary back, so I continued my research. Everything seemed to point to immunotherapy as the newest, most hopeful breakthrough in cancer treatment. And it made such perfect sense to me.

If the human body has a control factor for limiting the growth of cells, it would logically be contained within the immune system, which protects the body from foreign invaders like bacteria and viruses by producing antibodies which destroy them. It made sense that the immune system fights the body's own abnormal cells and that cancer is the result of a breakdown in our immunological defenses.

I read that any number of things could cause such a breakdown—an excess of drugs or hormones in the body, pollutants in the air, an excess of x-rays, poor diet. Some doctors were interested in the vitamin theory. They believed that our immune systems become screwed up because we eat so poorly. All the processed foods lacking in nutritional value, the over-abundance of preservatives and additives, the massive amounts of sugar.

Finally I felt I had learned all I needed to know in order to make a decision about taking BCG. I was convinced that immunotherapy must have tremendous value.

BCG, the anti-TB vaccine, simply got the defenses in

the immune system working. This tubercle bacillus, which is derived from cattle, is watered down so that it no longer is capable of causing tuberculosis. When it is injected into the body, the antibodies of the blood spring into action, attacking the BCG, a foreign agent. The tremendous buildup of antibodies caused by the presence of the BCG serves to repair the immune system, thereby destroying the cancer cells.

It sounded so simple, but I was certain there must be more to it. So I decided to speak with some oncologists before even trying to get into the Department of Oncology at UCLA. I wanted to make sure I understood perfectly what I was getting into.

I opened the phone book and started making appointments with doctors. I called and told the receptionists that I didn't want to be examined, I just wanted to confer with the doctors and that I'd pay for a full hour's consultation, just to get some information and advice.

The first appointment was with an oncologist in Beverly Hills. The day of the appointment, I organized all the articles I had on BCG and sat at the kitchen table going through each one, trying to figure out how I would present all the information to the Beverly Hills doctor. If he was anything like some of the other doctors I'd run across in the past eight years, he might know nothing about it.

David came into the kitchen and stood in front of the refrigerator, his favorite place. "Where's the apple juice, Mom? We out?"

I looked up briefly and then went back to my papers. "I think we are, David," I said absent-mindedly.

He shut the door with a firm shove and muttered, "Thanks a lot." He got a glass of water.

"Hmmmm?"

"Why didn't you get the apple juice while you were at the store?"

Briefly the old guilt flared. Then I got angry. "David,

how dare you yell at me the other night about making you feel guilty for not taking out the trash? Do you realize that I have spent most of my life feeling guilty for not doing this or that for you boys and your father?

"So what's the big deal about apple juice, I want to know? So I forget. You get an allowance. And you're seventeen years old. Going on eighteen already. From now on, I expect the trash outside the door on Thursday mornings by no later than seven o'clock. And if you're out of apple juice, I expect you to go buy some.

"Right now I'm busy trying to save my life. It may seem odd to you, David, but I do have my own life to live. And for the next few months, I may not have time to wipe your nose or spoon-feed you or buy you apple juice. So forgive me already."

I went back to my papers, aware that David was staring at me as if I were a freak. His mother was coming back to life. He'd never met his grandfather, but that day he saw a little of Papa sitting right at the kitchen table.

# Chapter 15

I SAW THIRTY-ONE DOCTORS in two weeks before I decided for sure that BCG was the treatment I wanted. I went from Beverly Hills to Century City to downtown Los Angeles to Culver City, from swank to not-so-swank to downright dismal offices, just to ask oncologists what they knew about immunotherapy and BCG.

It isn't what they told me that made me decide, it's what they didn't tell me. It's what I learned about doctors in general that made me decide I wanted to try the treatment.

If nothing else, my thirty-one doctor visits confirmed Papa's old saying about doctors being like other men. Many of them treated me with kindness and sympathy— the way you expect to be treated when you go to a doctor. But others treated me like a nut, a little stupid and slightly hysterical. Most of the doctors I visited during those two weeks seemed threatened by the new information I brought to their offices. They weren't ready for it.

Some just got mad at me. The audacity of this woman to think she knew as much as a doctor!

"Come back when you've had ten years of medical school and we'll discuss this, Mrs. Wallin," is the way one doctor closed our conversation.

"Everyone thinks he's a doctor!" said another, throwing up his hands.

"If you know so much about it, why are you asking me?" said some.

"Let me give you some books," offered others.

And, "I may not have all the answers, but I certainly have more than you do, Mrs. Wallin," was a familiar tune.

But I didn't think I knew it all. Maybe my cocky attitude put them off; I don't know. I had to psych myself up for each visit and present my case with a confidence I didn't always feel.

A couple of doctors were very sincere in their convictions that I was chasing wild dreams. They kept trying to convince me that chemotherapy was the only way to go. They said they wanted to see me live, and that I'd surely die if I took anything other than cobalt or chemotherapy.

After some of the consultations, I'd go home not so sure of myself. Maybe I *was* nuts. Maybe I'd better just travel the old familiar road. What if I tried BCG and died from the treatment? What if it had some fatal side effects they hadn't found out about yet? What if ten years later they discovered BCG was just a flash in the pan?

Every night I went home and studied the articles on BCG to reaffirm my convictions. What were the results of BCG on cancer patients?

"A woman dying of a massive, spreading breast cancer has been brought back from the dead by injections that included a vaccine derived from BCG."

"Three terminal cancer cases—people given only weeks or months to live by specialists—have been cured by BCG and are alive and healthy as long as eleven years later."

"Mrs. Marion Smythe, 70 years old, is one of a number of people alive today who were doomed to die of cancer, before Dr. Ray Villasor treated them with BCG."

I wanted to be one of the miracle cases. So I kept going back to doctors for more feedback. I was looking for just one doctor to say, "It sounds logical to me. It could work. Why don't you try it?" But few of them expressed even the remotest interest in it.

Several doctors tried to get me to come into their care. One of them changed his mind when he found out I didn't live in the posh Pacific Palisades where he practiced. When he found out I lived in the old dog-eared part of Culver City, he told me I should find a doctor in my area. The doctor was assuring himself of a paid bill, I guess.

I almost went on an all-out campaign against doctors for a while, muttering under my breath when the subject of doctors came up, throwing out sarcastic remarks whenever I got the chance, giving a lot of them a piece of my mind.

My bitterness didn't end until I finally realized that Papa's little saying about "a man like other men" included the fact that these doctors were entitled to be human, just like all other men.

Doctors set up practice after long years of medical school. They have families, civic duties, hobbies, social functions to attend, their own tragedies to cope with. Some of them don't have time to keep up with the latest developments in their fields. They treat patients in good faith with what they know to be available.

But I'd become convinced that one day immunotherapy would be one of their alternatives. On the other hand, I couldn't wait that long. If I could become a part of the experiment, I thought, maybe I could help hurry things along a little. And come out alive in the end.

# Chapter 16

So I DECIDED to try BCG. But I knew that it was only being used on melanoma patients at that time and that I might not even be able to get into the UCLA program, because I had carcinoma, not melanoma.

My main concern was getting into the inner sanctum at UCLA—the melanoma research program. I knew I could get into the oncology department, but the other might take some doing.

But I would do it. It was a terrific challenge. And I remembered how Papa always defied red tape and established procedure to get what he wanted.

I was a human being who deserved a chance. And I just wasn't going to listen this time to doctors like Dr. Hemp and Dr. Eisen who would say, "Let's wait" and "It's too experimental."

I didn't know exactly how to get a foot in the door at UCLA, but I knew I'd have to have a referral. I made an appointment with Dr. Eisen to talk it over with him.

As usual, he thought I was nuts. But he gave me the referral and even called UCLA and talked to a doctor in the oncology department there to tell them he was sending a patient to them.

I set off for UCLA on a steel gray January morning, with rain pouring down in buckets. I had wanted to race to the clinic but decided against it. What with the slippery streets and everything, it would be just too ironic if I had an accident on the way to the doctor.

I was determined to remain calm. I was not going to let them classify me as an hysterical woman who didn't know what she was talking about. I had even worn something appropriate—my one and only two-piece suit. It was navy blue and made me look rather worldly, I thought. Maybe it would give me credibility, but above all, I would be calm. I would be calm. *I would be calm.*

I entered the huge medical complex and followed the white line to the elevators that would take me to the seventh floor. Papa's words raced through my mind all the way up. Rules were made to bend and break. Go to the top. Fight for what's worthwhile. Calm. Calm. Calm.

When the doors opened I lunged through them, not exactly a calm exit, and practically bowled over a lady who was waiting to board. I apologized profusely and stopped myself from falling by grabbing the wall behind me. My knees threatened to crumple, and I told myself to slow down. I knew I had to calm myself, to clear my mind, and I was thankful for the slight accident that had forced me to slow down. I fought the cold fear that filled me and stepped away from the wall. I took a deep breath and walked into the reception room, clutching my medical files and x-rays as if they were some life-sustaining apparatus that would shut off my breathing if I let go of them.

I went through all the procedures—spoke with the receptionist, filled out some forms, took them back to the receptionist, went over the questionnaire with her, answered a few questions, handed her my medical file, and then went back to my seat to wait.

It seemed like hours. I tried to look through a few magazines, but my mind was racing with all the things I'd say to the doctor. I was there for BCG, which I had researched thoroughly after becoming familiar with it through an article I had read in the *National Enquirer*. There was no reason I shouldn't be admitted to such an experimental program, if it was my own choice. I was willing to participate. I was doing them a favor. I felt immunotherapy was a logical way of treating cancer and wanted to see if it would work in my own body. If it would work on carcinoma as well as melanoma, it might be an even greater breakthrough. Calmly he would say thank you, that he was grateful I had chosen to become part of the program.

My name was called. I stood up, felt dizzy, and had to sit down again. I got up and marched to the examining room, where I was told to undress for an examination.

"You know, honey, I'm really not here for an examination," I told the nurse. "All I want to do is talk to the doctor for a few minutes and then if he wants to examine me . . ."

"Mrs. Wallin, I'm afraid you'll have to let the doctor examine you before he can prescribe treatment for you. It's procedure."

Procedure, I told myself, was a bunch of bullshit. But I smiled and took the hospital gown. I'd sacrifice this fight to win the battle.

The doctor was young—too young, I told myself the minute he walked in the door. My mind was working out strategies. Should I appeal to him as mother to son, should I flatter him, cajole him, plead with him, be curt and businesslike, or what? I realized that I was shaking like a leaf as he flipped wordlessly through the pages of my file.

He was dark, bearded, and handsome. Maybe I should appeal to his masculinity. Probably had an ego as big as the clinic. But you couldn't tell. I'd wait and let him talk first.

His skill was apparent in the way he used his hands, searching for the lymph nodes. After he had probed for a while, he said softly, "Where does the pain seem to be centered?"

"Everywhere," I replied. Too passionately. Don't get excited, Bernice, I told myself.

"Does it stop with the pain killers?"

"Yes. Sometimes." Then, I don't know, it was like I had no control over my mouth. I blurted out, "Doctor, I came here specifically to be treated with BCG. I've studied it thoroughly, read everything I could find on the subject, and I'd like to be part of your research program. I think it could help me."

Damn it! I'd wanted to be so poised. Instead I had sounded like a tape recording on high speed. It had definitely been the wrong approach. He was staring at me with a frown all over his face.

"Mrs. Wallin, you couldn't know more than we do here about immunotherapy and we don't know that much. I really don't see how it could be warranted in your case."

"Why not?" All semblance of confidence left me and I had begun to whine. But I couldn't help it. I had planned this meeting so carefully and thought I would be prepared to argue. But I was already near tears, listening to the sound of defeat from a man young enough to be my own son.

"Well, first of all, we're only giving it to melanoma patients right now."

"I know that," I said. "But you can't tell me that melanoma and carcinoma are so far removed from each other that it's impossible for BCG to work in my case."

"Not impossible, no, nothing's impossible, but we have to . . ."

"Look, if you can immunize against melanoma, you can immunize against any other kind of cancer. If BCG is used to stop the spread of melanoma cancer cells, then it could do the same for my metastasis. True?"

"You're talking in hypothetics, and 'could be' is not the issue here. You don't qualify for BCG because you don't have melanoma, and that's just the way it is, Mrs. Wallin. We can't to give everyone whatever they ask for when they come in here. We have rules we have to go by."

"Rules? What kind of rules?"

"The rules that govern our grants," he replied.

I hadn't been ready for this argument. Of all the arguments I'd imagined, this one had never entered my mind. "Wait a second, what do you mean? Explain."

"Our research is funded by government grants, Mrs. Wallin, and in order to maintain those grants, we have to provide certain statistics. This particular grant is given to us so we can experiment with the effects of BCG on melanoma patients. You cannot be part of the research, because you don't have melanoma."

Now I was mad. "You mean to tell me that even if BCG, which I have read is giving fantastic, miraculous results, could save my life, I can't have it because I won't fit into your statistics?"

"That's absolutely correct."

"Oh, I see. The government dictates my treatment. Not the doctors. Not me. The government."

The doctor just stood there, but he looked kind of sorry. "I'm just telling you the way it is," he said. "Now if the pain gets too bad, there are ways we can go that have proven effective in many cases."

"I don't want any of those treatments!" I yelled at him. "Those treatments are bullshit treatments."

"Look, Mrs. Wallin, now don't get . . ."

I bit my tongue. "Sorry. Sorry. I've just been through this a million times with a million doctors, and I don't want any poison circulating around in my body. My body is in bad enough shape without any of that crap making things worse. Listen. Doctor: Will you tell me something? Isn't it possible it could help? I'm not saying is it possible for me to get into your program. But is it possible for BCG to be effective against all cancer it it's effective with melanoma patients?"

"I'm sorry, Mrs. Wallin. I don't know."

"Okay. Okay. That's all I wanted from you, doctor."

I got dressed and stomped, as best as I could with my limp, back out to the reception room. I was not going to be defeated. On the contrary, this setback spurred me on. I stopped at the reception desk and asked for another appointment. "And not with the same doctor," I told the receptionist. "I want another doctor. A little older, if you can. And one with more authority than that one, if it can be arranged."

She didn't tell me who it would be, the next doctor, but she put me down for the following week.

I waited the week nervously. I read day and night, brushing up on my plan of attack. Maybe the next doctor would listen to me if I were a little more convincing. That federal grant restriction—that was just a rule. And rules were meant to bend and break. I couldn't let a little thing like the government stand in my way.

The next doctor's visit was not as traumatic. This time I was calmer. The doctor had a new argument, but it was one I'd anticipated. This was an experimental program, he told me, and they were taking a big enough chance with the melanoma patients; taking a new kind of patient into the program was a risk they couldn't afford to take.

"But I'm the one who's taking the risk," I explained logically. "And I'm willing to do that. It's my life we're experimenting with, and I'm glad to let you experiment with it."

But he didn't accept my argument and the visit ended the way the first visit had ended. No. We can't put you in the program.

Still I was undaunted. I made another appointment and

again I told the receptionist that I wanted a more experienced doctor with a little more authority—one who really might have the power to do something with my case if I could convince him to do so.

But the third and fourth appointments were equally unsuccessful. Still, I hadn't given up, though I was beginning to worry. I made a fifth appointment, with a doctor who was a woman. Maybe she would be more compassionate, I thought. Maybe I could appeal to her woman to woman. Perhaps she'd be able to empathize with the plight of a woman who'd had a double mastectomy and a hysterectomy and was trying to save what was left of her body.

My will to live had altered my feelings about those earlier surgeries. Although in 1966 and 1967, I had been resigned about the mastectomies, my feelings had changed through the years. It wasn't that I felt the loss of my breasts would be a deterrent to a future relationship. And it wasn't that I felt that I had been mutilated by the breast surgery. It was just that sometimes I wished I still had 'em.

There were moments when I pined over not being able to wear plunging necklines and tight sweaters. And the stupid bras designed for mastectomy patients were anything but helpful. They were light-weight inflatable things that kept riding up around the neck or slipping down around the waist. I always had to sew pieces of elastic to the bottom of the bra and pin them to my slacks to keep the bra from slipping. Made me feel like a freak. Made me feel lousy as hell. I had begun to care about my appearance.

When I kept my fifth appointment, I was amazed to find that I didn't have to appeal to her as a woman after all. She skimmed through my files, did the probing, and then told me in a matter-of-fact tone that she had found some nodes in my neck and under my arm. "Mrs. Wallin, they will have to be removed before you can have BCG." I nearly fell off the examining table.

"What?" I gasped. I remembered immediately the

dreadful significance of lymph nodes in the body.

"When cancer is in your nodes, the cancer cells are probably throughout your entire body. They'll have to be removed before BCG can be administered."

"You mean if I have them removed I can have BCG?" I almost leaped off the table and threw my arms around her like a little kid who had been told she could stay up late and watch her favorite TV program.

"Have them removed and come back and then we'll see," was all she said.

So I went to see my surgeon, Dr. Meadows, feeling quite victorious. He examined me, felt the nodes, and said, "Bernice, these aren't malignant nodes. Why would they want you to have them removed? It's unnecessary surgery."

I was stubborn, though. I told him that if I had them removed, there was a possibility I might receive BCG at UCLA. The doctor was aware of what was being done with BCG, and he informed me that there was no correlation between these nodes and BCG treatments.

But what did he know, I reasoned. He wasn't over there doing the experiments. I didn't say that to him, but I simply insisted I wanted them removed. So he scheduled me for out-patient surgery at Mt. Sinai Hospital.

David drove me to the hospital since I would be unable drive after the surgery. I was in a great mood—babbled all the way to the hospital about how when you want something you have to stick to it and never give up.

The surgery was painful, despite the anesthetic I received. I felt the surgical instrument slash my neck and the blood gush out. It was a terrible feeling. I begged for more sedation, but to no avail.

Before leaving the hospital, the surgeon told me that the nodes were indeed benign as he had told me they would be, and he repeated his dismay over having to remove them. But what did he know, I repeated to myself. Despite my discomfort over the surgery, I was in a pretty good state of mind.

I left Mt. Sinai looking a little like a mummy, bandaged from the top of my neck to below my arms, my right arm sticking out stiffly from my side.

I recuperated at home in a joyful state of mind, anticipating with eagerness my return to that marvelous doctor who was going to see to it that I was given BCG. Three days before the appointment, most of the bandages were removed and I felt great.

But when I went back to UCLA, she wasn't there anymore. She had gone on to Michigan or someplace to continue her studies—probably in home economics or something.

I was given another doctor, one I hadn't seen before. He asked me why I was bandaged around my neck and I explained that the reason I was bandaged was that I was going to be admitted to the BCG program but first had to have some nodes removed.

"Who told you that you were going to be admitted to the BCG project?" he wanted to know.

I told him, my defenses to the forefront, trying to remain cool and calm.

"Well, that doctor has left UCLA, Mrs. Wallin, and I see nothing here in your chart about her telling you she was going to try to get you into the BCG project. I can't imagine her telling you such a thing. With the widespread metastasis you have, BCG would have no effect whatsoever."

"Now wait a minute, I'm telling you she said there was a possibility I could get into the program if I had these nodes removed. I don't care what it says there, that's what she told me."

"Why would she tell you that? Look, a one-centimeter malignancy contains one billion cancer cells, and that kind of malignancy in your body has already outstripped the immune response."

In all the reading I had done, never once had I found that cancer could possibly outstrip a properly working immune system. The whole BCG theory depended on the fact that a properly working immune system would fight off any foreign invaders in the body. I told him what I'd read.

"Well, I know you've probably read a lot, but so have I, Mrs. Wallin, and I promise you, with the four-centimeter tumor in your hip bone, you have four times the maximum amount BCG can help. And besides that, the node in your rib could also contain a billion or more cancer cells. Who knows how many more are circulating through your system? That's just too much for BCG to handle."

Well, it was the first definite approach any doctor at UCLA had taken with me. Before it had been rules and grants and statistics, too experimental, the wrong kind of cancer. Now the problem was that I had too much cancer for BCG to take care of. And the doctor seemed to know what he was talking about. How could I fight that?

I couldn't even get angry about the fact that I had gone through painful surgery only to hear that I was too far gone to get what I'd been fighting so hard to get. I was too stunned, too shaken.

David drove me home, and I cried all the way. Big deep sobs—I almost drove David to distraction. "Mom. Stop. It's going to be okay. Please stop."

But I didn't stop. I kept bawling through the rest of the afternoon, face down on my bed. When I was too exhausted to cry any longer, I dozed off.

It was dark when David came tiptoeing back into the room. "Mom," he whispered. "Are you okay?"

I rolled over, weak from crying. "Yeah," I said sullenly.

David had a package with him, which he handed to me. "I got you something," he told me. "Just something I thought you might like to have. I heard you talking to Lillian on the phone the other day. And I thought this would . . . Well, I thought you might like to have this."

I sat up in bed and took the paper bag he handed me. "What is it, David?"

He got up and backed out of the room "Just open it and

try it on and see if you can use it," he said, leaving me alone, switching on the overhead light and closing the door behind him.

In the bag I found a bra. It was the kind I had discussed with my friend Lillian, another mastectomy patient. It was a skin-like plastic form filled with glycerin, and it had a foam rubber backing to keep it from irritating the skin. I sat and looked at it, not knowing whether to laugh or cry.

I tried it on and it fit. It was almost exciting to have it on. I ran and pulled out a couple of things I hadn't been able to wear for years because they had to be tucked into my pants or skirts. And I could wear them again. Not bad. That son of mine.

I walked weakly out into the living room to thank him, but he had some of the band members over and I didn't want to embarrass him. I just smiled at him and he smiled back. I sat down and chatted a few minutes with the boys, then leaned back on the sofa and listened to them talk about their lives. Their nice, healthy, normal lives.

Then I started feeling like a slob. The way I'd let the house go. It was embarrassing to have people in my house when it looked like a pig sty. Of course they were David's friends, and it didn't seem to bother him enough to do anything about it. But it was my responsibility, I told myself, and guilt caught me at a weak moment, so I went into the kitchen and pulled out a mop. I started mopping the floor, which was so dirty it was sticky in spots and turned the mop black. I scrubbed and rinsed and scrubbed some more. Soon I heard the familiar refrain of "Johnny B. Goode" coming from the den. The band was practicing. It was one of my favorites, and I started to hum as I mopped the floor. The beat was driving and lifted my spirits a little. What's more, the bra was nice. It moved with me instead of away from me.

The music sounded so good that I started mopping in time to the beat and throwing in a few fancy steps.

Then, when they got into "Blue Suede Shoes," I threw

down the mop and started jitterbugging across the kitchen floor, out into the living room and down into the den. I was stark raving mad, I guess, but it made the boys in the band laugh and they started to play even faster.

The drummer dropped his drumsticks and joined me. He did the latest dance steps and I jitterbugged around him. Everyone was laughing and having a good time, but I was having the best time of all. It had been years! But I remembered how.

When the music stopped, my partner fell on the floor, exhausted. I was pretty beat, but I wasn't panting; he was. In fact, I was ready to go another round. He was too tired, so David danced with me. After I'd had a turn with each of the band members, I gave up and fell into the rocking chair, laughing. It was the most fun I'd had in years.

The next morning I called Oncology at UCLA and told the receptionist I wanted to speak with the head of the department.

"Dr. Morton? I'm afraid Dr. Morton doesn't see patients, ma'am. He has a schedule of . . ."

"I have a complaint to take up with Dr. Morton," I said, with a stroke of genius. He might not see me to discuss my cancer, but he'd have to answer for this idiot doctor who told me to get unnecessary surgery. "Now one of your doctors there made a damn big mistake with me and I want to know what's going on over there. One hand doesn't seem to know what the other hand is doing, and I intend to take it up with the person who is in charge, whoever that may be. If Dr. Morton doesn't want to talk to me, maybe somebody else will."

She made an appointment for me to see Dr. Morton. Finally, I was at the top. Why had I bothered with anyone else in the first place?

I took David to the office with me—to see how a battle is won. I had a little something to hold over their heads, and I wasn't going to be denied this time.

Dr. Morton was a big man, but he didn't look threatening. He was rather a mild-mannered, shy fellow, actually.

He quietly went through the preliminaries and then asked what my specific complaint was.

I told him about the doctor who had told me that I could have BCG if I had the nodes removed. He said he was terribly sorry, but that she had been a new doctor in the UCLA oncology department and had evidently not been informed that he was the one who made decisions as to what patients were to be admitted to that treatment.

I seized on that and began explaining to him why I should be admitted.

He voiced every objection I'd heard in the past. This time I was ready for them. I spoke calmly, with confidence and conviction. And I realized that all the other doctors I'd seen before were simply the training ground for this meeting, this very important meeting which would determine whether or not I'd be allowed to enter the BCG program.

He was negative for almost an hour. I hung on as long as I could. Finally it looked like the session was over. I'd taken an hour of the good doctor's time, and he stood up, looking at his watch and telling me that he was terribly sorry, but . . .

I used the final ammunition. I cried. Not that I had to force myself. I was desperate, and I saw my chance slipping away.

"Now Mrs. Wallin, I know how you feel. I know how you feel."

"You don't know how I feel," I cried. "Doctors don't know how their patients feel. That's the whole problem. I want to live. People with cancer don't make it with chemotherapy. They die. Look at your statistics, if you're so interested in statistics. If BCG is helping people, then I want some."

He sighed and sat back down in his chair, just staring at me as I wiped the tears away and sobbed quietly.

Finally he said the words. "Okay. Okay, we'll try you on it."

I looked up at him. "You will?"

"Look, I don't like the idea. But I have to agree with you in one regard, Mrs. Wallin. You're entitled. You're entitled to try something that may save your life. But I want you to remember that I said *may*. Is that understood? Because before I go into this treatment with any of my patients, I explain that to them. There are only incomplete statistics at this point and there are no promises made here. Are you clear on that?"

I nodded.

Then he made me sign a paper and David, having just turned eighteen, proudly signed as my witness. I don't know if he was proud because he was old enough to sign or proud because he had just seen his mother win something she'd been fighting long and hard to get.

Dr. Morton explained to me that the last doctor I had seen was correct when he told me that some immune systems were too far depressed to be receptive to BCG and that skin-testing would show us whether or not this was true in my case.

But for some reason I wasn't worried about that. Skin-testing seemed like nothing compared to the test I had just been through.

# Chapter 17

IT WAS TESTING TIME AGAIN—the familiar bone, brain, and liver scans, the lying on tables, the uncomfortable positions, the endless waiting.

But the important tests were the skin tests they took to check the functioning of my immune system. One set of tests determined my present immune response, while another set determined my past immune history. Blood was drawn for antibody tests to determine my body's immune response to the malignancy. These tests would tell whether or not I was a candidate for the BCG program. And after they were taken, I had to wait sixteen days for the results.

Those sixteen days seemed longer to me than any of the other waiting periods I'd had to go through. I tried not to talk about it at home or to my friends. I mean, there's only so much a person wants to hear about another person's state of health. But I dreamed about it, thought about it, fantasized getting my health back. If the BCG worked, and if I got well, oh boy, the things I would do.

Finally the waiting period was over and I went to UCLA for the results. I sat on the treatment table as if I were sitting in the audience at the Academy Awards to see if I'd won an Oscar. What kind of acceptance speech would I make? If I lost, how would I take it?

"Your immune system is functioning at a very weak level, Mrs. Wallin," the doctor told me. My heart missed a beat. Go on. Go on. "But it is functioning. And we've decided to admit you to the program."

I felt like standing up and taking a bow. Thank you, ladies and gentlemen, thank you. And now for my encore, I'm going to regain my health.

That same day I received my first BCG treatment. I put on the white hospital gown in the same state of mind in which I'd put on my wedding gown. Nervous as a virgin bride. Anticipating . . . dreading.

The nurse came in carrying a stainless steel tray covered with a white cloth on which were scattered a few instruments. She explained the procedure as she went along. The main item, she told me, was a *tine,* a ¾-by-1-inch rectangular piece of metal. Inside it there were nine squares with four prongs on each of the corners, making a total of thirty-six prongs. Each prong was 2 millimeters long. A magnet was attached to the part she was holding in her hands, which were gloved in thin, white translucent plastic. She told me that the BCG would be applied to four areas of my body near the lymph glands—on both sides of the breast area and on either side of the groin area. The lymph glands would pick up and distribute the solution throughout my system. In order to remove the body oils, she rubbed acetone on the four areas to be injected. Then she dropped three or four drops of BCG from a syringe onto each of the four sites of my body and rubbed it lightly. She took the tine and punctured each of the four areas twice, penetrating intradermally ⅛-inch under the skin, for a total of 288 punches. "Ouch!" I said each time the needles pricked my skin. It hurt for an instant and then the pain was gone.

I kept chattering away, asking her questions. Did she know anyone who had been cured with this treatment? Well, she said, it had been very helpful in controlling melanoma in many instances, but she didn't know that much about breast-cancer, metastisized patients. She said there were many patients engaged in this program. I asked her where the BCG came from, and she said it was shipped to UCLA from the University of Illinois in freeze-dried ampules, and diluted with one cubic centimeter of sterile water, no preservatives. Each ampule treated two patients.

After the BCG treatment was over, the nurse told me to wait five or ten minutes to allow the injected areas to dry before getting dressed. She gave me a piece of cardboard to fan the damp places. I wasn't to bathe or shower for forty-eight hours, she said, because it took that long for the BCG to be absorbed into the body.

About ten or twelve hours after the treatment, I experienced a slight headache, chills, an ache in my nose like a sinus pain, and a feeling of general fatigue. I felt as if I were coming down with a cold.

The areas that had been injected started to redden and swell in ten or twelve days. Tender sores appeared. Some of the sores blistered and broke open, making a sticky mess on my underwear. It ached and it itched and I had been told not to scratch. I was extremely uncomfortable. But when I weighed my discomfort against the possibility of a cure, it didn't seem so bad. In fact, I rejoiced. The sores were a sign that my immune system was reacting.

In March I received a letter from Fred in Boston. He enclosed an article printed in *Time* magazine which stated that Sloan Kettering Cancer Center in New York City was experimenting with BCG and that there was a Dr. Robert Good there who was especially enthusiastic about the results.

I telephoned the Sloan Kettering Center and spoke to an oncologist in the Breast Cancer Clinic. I explained my particular case and asked if there was anything they had to offer me that UCLA did not have. The doctor advised me to remain with UCLA because I was getting the same type of treatment they were giving at Sloan Kettering.

Fred had circled one of the paragraphs, which stated that BCG, unlike the other methods of cancer therapy, does not destroy normal cells in the body, and that it was unique in that it alone destroyed the residual cancer cells, leaving no potential cancer in the patient.

That statement gave me the hope and confidence I so badly needed.

Before each treatment, there were varied blood counts. One of them included the SMA-12 test, which determines the twelve chemistries of the blood and gives the doctor an almost overall picture of the functioning of the body. If one of the test results is above the normal limits, then added specific tests are ordered to determine where the trouble is.

I'd return home from these blood counts and treatments tired, irritable, and depressed. It wasn't the endless blood testing that exhausted me. Nor was it the countless scans, x-rays, or metastatic surveys. It was the horrible agony of waiting for the test results. Would this week's test show my cancer had gone a step further? Invaded another one of my organs? The waiting drove me practically out of my mind.

I'd stand in front of the doctor, trembling, my heart pounding wildly. If the report was satisfactory, I'd walk out of the office, return home, and throw myself into an orgy of house cleaning. When the reports were alarming, I'd revert to lying in my bed or I'd go to the beach and, stoned to the gills, I'd sit on a bench and watch people walk by. The reports pulled at my emotions like a string on a yo-yo.

The first year of the BCG treatments passed slowly. That year I felt I had aged twenty years. My body felt as if it had been completely swallowed by an ocean of pain. My time was spent waiting for the results of my tests and waiting for the next pain pill, and the indescribable relief it would bring.

On one of my first visits to UCLA, Dr. Frank Sparks told me that my cancer was spreading into the thighbone. A bone survey had shown a larger gray area on the x-ray film. I remember breaking down completely, sobbing hysterically in his office. That was one of the times I had come to UCLA alone. David was busy taking a college exam.

Dr. Sparks soothed and comforted me and gave me words of hope. God bless him.

The second year was the hardest. My pain was there most of the time unless I was heavily drugged on pain killers. At times I felt nearly defeated. I doubted that BCG treatments were even working. After all, the vaccine was experimental. There were not too many statistics to go by. The hardest part of that year was the waiting to see if BCG would work and the agony of waiting, day after day. I knew BCG would take time to work. I had to be patient. When the malignancy left my body, so would the pain.

There were a few weeks, during my illness, when the pain was unbearable. I started begging for cobalt, and that was something I'd promised myself I'd never resort to. Dr. Sparks talked me out of it by saying, "Bernice, please, let's wait a little while longer. Bear it. Let's see if BCG will take hold." I'm glad I followed his advice.

It wasn't always convenient for David to arrange his college schedule so that he could drive me to get my BCG. Sometimes there were classes and exams he couldn't afford to miss.

One day during that first year of treatments, David's station wagon wouldn't start and he asked me to drive him to school. I said that I would be glad to, but that first I had to go to UCLA for my treatment. His reaction surprised me.

"Great," he said. "I don't have to get to school until ten and you're always done before that. I'll go with you to see what those BCG shots are like."

My sons had lived in a house filled with cancer for so long that it was nothing for David to say something like that, but I didn't quite know how to take his enthusiasm. I was pleased by his concern but slightly taken aback by his zeal.

"Sure," I said and we drove to UCLA.

When David started to accompany me into the room where I got my shots, the nurse asked him to wait outside while she gave me my treatment. But I told her I wanted David to watch.

I studied David's expression as he watched the nurse administer the vaccine. When I said "Ouch" as the needles pricked my skin, it wasn't from the pain. David's face was white; it shocked me. His lips started to tremble. He didn't turn away and he tried not to wince, but I could see that it was hard for him.

I tried easing the situation. "David, it's not that bad. Really it isn't."

"That's not how it looks from here," he answered, between clenched teeth.

Usually we find a lot to gab about, David and I. His band, his new girlfriend, the books I'm reading, school. But we were silent as I drove him to school.

"What's the matter, Dave?" I asked.

"Mom, how can you stand taking those shots week after week? Wow, they must really hurt. I see you taking pain pills all the time. You don't even know if the BCG is helping you. Doesn't it drive you out of your mind?"

"Dave, they're not that bad. Sure it hurts some and it's uncomfortable a lot of the time, but if the shots might help, I'm going to keep taking them and hoping."

He bit his bottom lip as he answered, "Sure, yeah, I suppose you're right."

I parked at the curb to let him out. "David," I said, taking hold of his sleeve, "I don't like to go back to the subject of your brother Gary. We don't talk about him much anymore because I know it's depressing for you kids. But if I can stand the pain of losing Gary, I can just about stand any other kind of pain. Nothing can compare with how I hurt from missing Gary."

He put one foot out of the car and turned to me. "Mom, I hardly remember Gary," he said in a troubled voice.

"So you've got a lousy memory anyhow. You never know what day of the week it is. Now get to your class. You don't want to miss flirting with that sexy blonde who sits next to you, do you? I'm parked in the red. Skidoo."

As I turned the car around and drove away, he yelled, "Hey Mom, pick me up at two and don't be late."

One day the UCLA billing department sent me a letter stating that my account was going to be put into the hands of a collection agency unless it was paid in full. There was no question in my mind that the BCG treatments would be discontinued if this happened.

I considered getting a job and scanned the want-ads. I wanted to find something that wouldn't take too much concentration. Sitting for any length of time drove me buggy. I wanted a job where I could move about, despite the constant pain. In skimming through the classifieds, I found a job that was being offered by a catering company that prepared sandwiches daily. They wanted a person to sell their sandwiches door to door in Beverly Hills office buildings. The pay was lousy but they didn't seem to mind my age or the fact that I wasn't particularly vivacious.

I phoned the UCLA billing department and told them I had found a job and was going to be paying off my bill in short order. I was told that my account had already been placed in the hands of the collection agency and that there was nothing they could do about it.

Remembering Papa's philosophy of always going to the top, I dialed UCLA and asked to speak to the administrator of the hospital. In a matter of seconds, I was explaining my situation to the top man. The matter was resolved by my signing a promissory note and my BCG treatments continued uninterrupted.

I trudged my sandwich route five days a week from ten to one. It was a hell of a lot of painful walking, but I paid the note in full at the end of the year.

Many mornings after a treatment, I'd hobble to the biomedical library and search for more material on BCG. When some of the reports I read sounded negative, a funny weakness, beginning somewhere under my stomach, would engulf me. I'd close the book, pick up my belongings, and race home.

But despite the pain and the fear, I did derive some pleasure from my reading. I allowed it to absorb my complete attention so that my mind was not on my pain. And by doing that, I began to feel that I had a life apart from the life I shared with my family. I had my own world to retreat to and grow in. It was a weird, wonderful feeling. A whole new dimension of living. The unborn creature in me was stirring.

I remember one afternoon when I sat on the couch reading. I was not as involved in it as I usually was. My mind wandered. My thoughts jumped around and around. I started thinking about all the friends I had. I thought about how I might be heading toward death while they were all in relatively good health. And then I was struck by a very strange thought. Even if it were possible, I would not want to be any of my friends. I wouldn't want to be anyone but who I am. That thought startled me so much that it has affected my attitude from that moment to the present. A middle-aged woman, wrinkles and all, and I was at last moving toward completion.

Mama died during that second year. She was eighty-nine. I wished with all my heart that I had told her that I loved her. I wish death would leave a warning calling card for those of us who are thoughtless, so we could make some last minute amenities to alleviate the guilt feelings that linger for years after the death of a loved one.

Mama left the boys a little money. David decided to add on a soundproof room to the back of his bedroom so that his band could practice without disturbing our neighbors.

So it was chaos again, the chaos that goes with adding on a room. The sound of the cement truck grinding, the hammering, the sawing, the mess. David, some of his friends, and I did as much of the work as possible to hold the construction costs down. Helping David was great therapy for me. It kept me busy, kept my mind off the constant pain and kept me from dwelling on some rather frightening reports that kept coming out of UCLA concerning my brain scans. Requests were being made repeatedly for more extensive brain scans. My skull was beginning to show an irregular pattern.

"Not my brain!· Not my brain!" I prayed as I pounded on nail after nail.

"Hey Mom, not that hard," David would say, taking the hammer from me. "You'll knock yourself out."

The skull patterns continued to be irregular for a while, along with a strong suspicion that cancer could be there. But then gradually, *wonderfully,* the pain began to ease. I stopped taking so many pain killers. I went to bed a little later, got up a little earlier, and the time in between became clearer.

# Chapter 18

O<small>N A WARM SPRING DAY</small> in May 1975, the attending UCLA physician examined me, sat down on the stool on the other side of the room, and said, "Bernice, the last few tests we've done on you show that you don't have one trace of cancer in your body anywhere. The metastasis in your bone has disappeared. The nodule in your ribs is gone, and your skull is showing perfectly normal patterns."

The cancer was gone! I felt a powerfully warm sensation. I felt grateful. I would live to dance at Fred's and David's weddings. No trace of cancer. The news was like a pain killer. I couldn't believe that the cancer was gone. All those years of waiting for death began to fade away.

I followed the young intern out of the examining room. He had to get back to his patients. I had to get back to my life. But how could I believe the cancer was gone, not one trace?

That morning I went directly from UCLA to the Beth Olam Cemetery. Part of my reason for going, I know, was not to share gratitude but to suppress it, to put a damper on it. Gary was dead. How could it feel so wonderful to be alive? I let the guilt close around my joy.

I visited Papa's crypt out of respect before I went to Gary's. I felt good there. I felt a new sensation of gratitude, a deep one, to Papa. "Papa, you taught me the principles that made me fight for BCG and get it. I fought for my life and won. Thank you, Papa."

And then I thanked myself for saving my own life.

To Gary, I said, "But it is you, my son, that I thank with all my heart. Your life gave me mine."

I stood silently in front of Gary's crypt, looking up at the plaque bolted to the front of the marble plate. "Gary Arnold Wallin. Beloved son and brother, 1957–1965, *Victim of Leukemia.*"

I had wanted to declare to the world that Gary had been killed by that monstrous disease. Now I wanted to cry out to the world that what I had learned while Gary was dying had led me to UCLA, led me to BCG, years after Gary's death, when my own hung before me.

I think that was the moment, if there was such a moment, that the nucleus for this book was born.

On the way home from the cemetery, I tried to decide how to break the wonderful news. Should I blurt it right out to David and say, "Dave, everything's gone. Look at me. I'm not sick anymore"? No, I thought. I want to get the full effect. I'll take my time.

The door was open and I could hear David's guitar. The playing stopped when he heard my footsteps.

"Hi, Mom," he said, walking into the living room.

"Hi yourself."

I went into the kitchen to pour myself some apple juice and shouted into the living room. "Any phone calls?"

"Nope."

"Did you have lunch?" I came back into the living room and tousled his hair.

"Nope."

"Is that all you can say? 'Nope'?"

"Yup."

"Dave, have you seen our old tennis rackets around lately?"

"Nah. I haven't seen them for a long while. They're probably in the garage. How come?"

"Well, I thought I'd take a few lessons and become another Billie Jean King."

"Mom, you're weird. You haven't played tennis since you got sick. You can't play tennis now."

"Well, I'm not sick anymore, David. You're looking at a healthy lady."

"Is that what your tests showed?"

"Yep. That's right."

I tried to hold back the tears that were forming in my eyes. David put his arms around me and hugged me tightly. We both began to cry. David hugged me tighter. "We'll play tennis together, Mom."

I dialed Fred in Boston. He must have just walked into his apartment because he sounded a little out of breath when he answered the phone.

"Mom, it's good to hear from you. What's going on?"

He never knew if my calls would bring good news or bad, but he always sounded happy to hear my voice.

"Not much. Just thought I'd say hello and I wanted to ask you if there are any spots open in the 1976 Olympics."

"What spots?"

"For the marathon."

"Why the sudden interest?"

"Where do I enter?"

It was a moment before Fred answered. "Mom, are you trying to tell me something I should know?"

"You guessed it. I saw the doctor at UCLA this morning."

"And?"

"He said"—I paused—"that he couldn't find anything. That my tests were normal. I think I'm going to make it."

"Mom, that's wonderful. How do you feel?"

"Like a million bucks."

From the joy in his voice, I could see his smile three thousand miles away.

"Fred, I don't want to cut this short, but I have to call the skywriters. I want them to put a message in the sky in giant letters and I want to make sure they spell my name correctly."

We hung up laughing.

When I dialed Paul at work, the girl who answered the phone told me he was at the law library doing research. I told her to have him call me back. I walked into the kitchen for a glass of water and the phone rang. It was my sister Sally. My words tumbled over one another as I told her the good news.

"Gee, that's great, Bernice," she said. "You've been so brave. I don't know how you take it like you do—your having no breasts, I mean. I'd kill myself if I lost my breasts."

"Like hell you would, sister dear," I answered tartly. "Life is precious, damn precious. It's not so bad for me, Sally, when you consider that I came so close to the alternative."

And then I added, "Sally, do you know what W. C. Fields has inscribed on his tombstone?"

"No. What?"

"'All things considered, I'd rather be in Philadelphia.'"

I leaned back against the couch after we hung up and dozed off. The ringing of the phone awakened me. It was Paul.

"What's up, Mom? How's things?"

"Fine. What's with you?"

"I'm doing some research on a criminal case. When I see you over the weekend, I'll tell you about it."

"Sounds interesting. How's Sharon?"

"Just fine. You went for your shots today? What did the doctor say?"

"Well," I spoke slowly and paused at every word. "It looks like I'm going to be around for a while."

"It was good news, then, huh?"

"You better believe it. The doctor told me I can breathe freely now. There's no sign of anything anymore."

"That's fantastic! No, it's more than that. The BCG really did the trick." I could feel the emotion in his voice. "Take care, Paul. Say hello to Sharon."

"Mom, you're invincible and I love you."

"I love you, too, Paul."

Jack walked in a little after six with his usual, "Hi, hon, what's for dinner?" He hung up his jacket in the closet and walked into the den and turned on the TV.

"What smells so good?"

"Roast chicken and brown potatoes. Jack, do you know where the old tennis rackets are?"

He looked up from the *TV Guide*. "How should I know where they are? I don't play tennis. What do you want with tennis rackets, anyhow?"

"Well, I thought I'd play a little tennis. I think I picked up a few pounds."

"You're not supposed to be that active with your condition."

"I can be as active as I want now. The cancer's gone."

"You're kidding."

"No, I'm not kidding."

"When did you get the news?"

"This morning."

"That's great. That's really great."

"The doctor and I looked at my x-rays together. It's getting so I can almost read the x-ray film. He said . . ."

"All right. All right. Let me watch this program."

"You care more about TV than you do about my life."

"It's not that. But you're alive. What's there to talk about?"

For a while I was doubtful that my cancer was gone. It was a strange feeling, to say the least, not worrying about death, not worrying about what was going on inside my body. Would it come back? I mean, after all, the doctors had told me it was gone once before.

I made them write me an official letter at UCLA, stating that the cancer had disappeared. For proof to myself and to others. Who would believe it? I myself didn't believe it.

Now I wanted to do things and go places. I wanted to detrch myself from the barnacles that had attached themselves to me.

Not that I wasn't grateful for David's concern. But his protectiveness was strangling me. There were discussion groups and political meetings I wanted to attend. I didn't want David to have to sit through those or to have to drive me to meetings and pick me up later. He had his own life to live.

At first it was hard for David to ease his guard over me. He still wanted to go everywhere with me, because he didn't trust me behind the wheel.

I tried to convince him that it was the pain killers and tranquilizers that had made my driving so freaky. Now that I was taking so few, I told him, my driving would improve. I was quite capable now of being a careful and efficient driver.

But David was stubborn.

Finally, I said, "Look, David, I was driving ten years before you were born. Don't forget that. Get off my ass." And he did. I felt guilty being so harsh with him, but I no longer wanted to feel like an invalid who couldn't make it to the corner drugstore without help.

# Chapter 19

**N**OW THAT ALL MY FANTASIES about getting well had been realized, I started making notes about all the things I wanted to do. An exercise program, some extension classes at UCLA, some writing, and a healthier diet. I'd been reading about diets and nutritional therapy and I'd become convinced that proper nutrition could be beneficial in controlling and preventing cancer. I was determined to *stay* healthy.

What I was reading made sense to me—a healthy body is much more resistant to cancer. If a body is in excellent health, and all the cells are functioning well, the cancer cells, which many researchers say are found in humans at all times, will not be activated. Good nutrition was necessary to keep the cells healthy and functioning, to provide energy, and to build and repair tissues.

So I started looking around for a doctor who specialized in nutrition and I found one who had a controversial practice. I'd heard about this doctor from people who considered him a brave pioneer in medicine because of his stand on Laetrile, but I'd also read things about him that weren't so favorable.

I decided to take my chances. I got in my car and drove thirty miles to his office in Covina.

When I met Dr. Privitera, I was impressed. He had an air of confidence about him and a sincere manner. He was in his early thirties, and exuded health.

After he'd gone through my medical file, he said, "Your report says you're cancer free."

"But am I? That's the question," I said.

"What do you think?"

"Well, I do a lot of reading. That happens to be one of the things that saved my life," I told him. "I read about BCG and pushed into the melanoma research project at UCLA. Anyway, I know that cancer is a systemic disease and a person has to stay on top of it forever, or it comes back. Right?"

A slow smile spread across his face. "You know your disease then, don't you? I'm glad. So what are we going to do with you?"

"Well, I've been reading a lot about Laetrile and about diet. I know Laetrile did nothing for my son. He died of leukemia nine years ago, even after I tried him on Laetrile. But I wanted to find out more about it anyway."

"Mrs. Wallin, leukemia is a tough one," he said. "Any other cancer but leukemia is easier to deal with."

"Well, what do you think? What really causes cancer? Is it a breakdown of the immune system?"

"Yes. Yes, it's that in part, but it's even more than that. Malignancy is a disorder of protein metabolism and it's caused by an inadequate production or use of enzymes. There is a general consensus among us doctors who study nutrition that people with malignant tumors have deficiencies in their active pancreatic enzymes. So while cancer is basically a vitamin deficiency disease, it's also caused by a deficiency in these enzymes."

He explained that the enzymes and the immunological system of the body are influenced by diet. Processed foods, he told me, like white flour and sugar, or foods with preservatives and additives, weaken the immune and enzyme system.

"When people stopped eating the seeds of common fruits, cancer became more prevalent," he said. "There are societies, like the Hunzakuts in the Himalaya Mountains, where the incidence of cancer is almost nil. These people eat enormous amounts of apricot seeds and other foods containing nitrilosides, which we don't get in most of our diets today."

"And that's where Laetrile comes in?"

"Amygdalin is a common food substance found in these seeds. Laetrile is just concentrated amygdalin. A natural food substance. We call it Vitamin B17."

"But doctor, some people say it's poisonous to the system," I pointed out.

He shook his head and looked amused. "That's propaganda," he said. "Let me explain. When B17 comes in contact with cancerous cells, it releases cyanide in the body—but only enough to kill the bad cells. When B17 comes next to healthy cells, the chemical reaction is entirely different. It's a perfectly natural chemical process, Mrs. Wallin. It isn't poisonous unless you overdose yourself with it. But then, too much of anything can be fatal, can't it? Look, I can tell you, I take massive quantities of Laetrile as a preventive measure every day, and I haven't poisoned myself yet."

What he said sounded logical. "Look at the diseases—scurvy, pellegra, pernicious anemia, and rickets. All of those were found to be vitamin deficiency diseases."

The more he talked, the more sense it made to me. And I decided to try it. Besides, like Papa, I wanted to hedge my bets. If there was anything to it, I wanted to be right there.

Dr. Privitera gave me a special diet to follow and a long

list of vitamins I was to take. My diet was to consist of whole grains, frest fruits and vegetables, raw fruit and vegetable juices, no processed foods, and fish sparingly.

The doctor explained to me that beef and fowl use all the enzymes needed to fight the cancer cells produced in our bodies. Not only that, he said, but these meats have a high female-sex-hormone content. Most animals sold for commercial purposes have been injected with large amounts of these hormones and they are thought to cause cancer.

"Now remember, Mrs. Wallin," the doctor said, as I left his office. "This is a completely holistic approach to cancer. It is a combination of proper nutrition, Laetrile, vitamins, minerals, and enzymes. To depend on Laetrile alone is foolhardy. We hope the combination will help strengthen the immune system, so that a person can throw off his own disease."

The doctor's program was not a cinch. I had to take over a hundred pills a day, and I had to change my eating habits completely. There were times when I would have sold my soul for a buttered bagel and a Herskey kiss. But I felt I was on the right track, and it was a great feeling.

The next step was getting off the tranquilizers. Making the decision was easy. It was actually doing it that drove me up a wall.

I decided to stop cold turkey. One day I was popping a tranquilizer every other hour and the next day I dumped them all down the toilet.

In the daytime it was fairly easy. I just kept busy. When the craving became really bad, I got in the car and went shopping or visiting.

But at night as I lay in bed, I felt a painful hollowness in my stomach. I used to toss and turn all night long, shivering and sweating, my muscles jerking and twitching.

One evening it got so bad I was afraid it might be symptoms of cancer again. I'd been off the tranquilizers for two weeks and I wasn't feeling any better.

I'd heard on the radio that Synanon had a hot line for drug addicts. I called.

"I'm a middle-aged lady who's been on pain pills and tranquilizers a long time for cancer. I've stopped the pills and changed my diet and it's been two weeks already and I'm still going crazy. When does the craving stop, anyway? Does it ever stop?"

She told me that I had at least another month of withdrawal to go through. If I'd eliminated sugar from my diet, she said, I was probably having withdrawal symptoms from that too, since sugar is addictive.

It took almost two months, but I finally stopped craving the barbiturates, and now I'm entirely free of everything. Free of the drugs and free from cancer. Liberated at last.

Today I find myself a woman minus her youngest son and both her breasts, but I am alive. Not quite physically whole, but a complete woman.

It's hard to believe that anything real can be created through loss. But it can. At one time I thought breasts and children were synonyms for womanhood. But that's all predicated on the misconception of what it is to be a woman.

Gary died when he was only seven years old. I would like more than anything in the world to be able to say that his death served some magnificent purpose. But how can I say that his death served a purpose more than his life would have, had he lived?

Gary had a genius I.Q. Even more important, he had a heart full of love. There is no telling what such a combination might have done for mankind. I know how deeply he affected those around him during the seven short years he was alive. His absence has affected me still more deeply.

There will never be a moment when my heart will not ache over the loss of my son. There will never be a moment when my heart will not pound furiously with anger that a control for leukemia could not have come soon enough for Gary.

Yet I have so much to be grateful for. Right now, I'm a very busy lady. I play tennis, ride my bike, play volleyball, and jog. I'm active in "Mastectomy Recovery Plus," a self-help breast cancer project organized in 1974. The group's goals are, primarily, the sharing of medical information and psychological support. I answer phone calls day and night from people who need advice on cancer treatments. Some of the stories I hear are familiar, because I've been there myself. But hearing about the tragedy and torture cancer brings never fails to make me both angry and heartbroken. All I can do is tell people how I beat cancer and hope they'll have the *chutzpah* to stick it through until they see the light of victory.

There are moments when I feel I would like to see if I could stand completely on my own two feet, both physically and emotionally. I'd like to discontinue the BCG treatments. With my diet and the care I'm taking with my health, my immune system should be able to function on its own. But then, my better judgment comes into play. "That's foolish, Bernice." I say. "Why press your luck?"

When I question the doctor about how long I will have to stay on the BCG vaccine, his answer is always the same. "Bernice, your guess is as good as mine. We're making medical history together."

So I'll continue the BCG treatments for now, but I have them only once a month, instead of once a week. I still have to take tests, suffer through biopsies, but I cope. I cope just fine. Now when I go to sleep and when I wake up, I can think of a tomorrow. And I expect to live without fear of that word. Because Bernice will definitely be around tomorrow.

One thing I've learned from my experiences is how ridiculous it is for people to accept their own death. They go to a doctor for help, get wheeled into a hospital, and never even bother to ask questions. They just accept what the doctors say and then they die.

They never try to find out about their disease themselves. They leave it all in the hands of the doctor and, believe me, he doesn't know it all.

Long before I read it, Papa was telling me, "Knowledge is power. What you don't know can hurt you and what you do know can only help you."

My sons are doing fine. Fred is hosting a local radio sports talk show and he's a freelance sportswriter. Paul graduated from law school, *cum laude*. Recently he took the bar exam and is awaiting the results. David's band is active. Wherever he's performing you will find me. He has a college degree in criminology, but he's determined to make it big in the entertainment world.

Now I have a future, too. I'm going back to school to take some public health classes. I'd love to work in preventive medicine, perhaps as a counselor, passing along some of my experiences to other people.

I think I may just get to enjoy life again, for the first time in thirteen years. According to a survey I read in either *Playboy* or *Penthouse,* men are far more interested in a woman's behind than in her breasts. Thank God, I still have my fanny.

And Papa, wherever you are, I think I'm going to do some dancing.